Liberating Medicine

David Seedhouse
Unit for the Study of Health Care Ethics,
Department of General Practice,
The University of Liverpool, UK

JOHN WILEY & SONS
Chichester · New York · Brisbane · Toronto · Singapore

Other Wiley Editorial Offices

John Wiley & Sons, Inc., 605 Third Avenue,
New York, NY 10158-0012, USA

Jacaranda Wiley Ltd, G.P.O. Box 859, Brisbane,
Queensland 4001, Australia

John Wiley & Sons (Canada) Ltd, 22 Worcester Road,
Rexdale, Ontario M9W 1L1, Canada

John Wiley & Sons (SEA) Pte Ltd, 37 Jalan Pemimpin 05-04,
Block B, Union Industrial Building, Singapore 2057

Library of Congress Cataloging-in-Publication Data
Seedhouse, David
    Liberating medicine / by David Seedhouse.
      p. cm.
    Includes bibliographical references.
    Includes index.
    ISBN 0 471 92844 5
    1. Medicine—Philosophy. I. Title.
    [DNLM: 1. Philosophy, Medical. W 61 S451L]
  R723.S44 1990
  610'.1—dc20
  DNLM/DLC
  for Library of Congress   90-12515
                           CIP

British Library Cataloguing in Publication Data
Seedhouse, David
  Liberating medicine.
  1. Medicine. Ethical aspects
  I. Title
  174.2

ISBN 0 471 92844 5

Phototypeset by Dobbie Typesetting Limited, Tavistock, Devon
Printed and bound by Courier International, Tiptree, Colchester

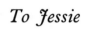

To Jessie

'What has this got to do with me? I'm going to be a doctor.' Medical student, Great Britain 1989—following a lecture on the influence of ethics, law and economics on medicine.

Contents

Foreword

The capacity of medicine to intervene in the lives of people has increased enormously during the 25 years of my professional career. This increase stems not only from significant technical advances but also from the declared scope of certain branches of the profession (such as my own) which now recognise *psychological* and *social* as well as *physical* dimensions of health and illness. Understandably, this has excited comment, usually from outside the profession, by critics who fear misapplied technology and intrusive intervention. Some of this fear has rubbed off onto the general public who, while respectful of medicine's achievements, are becoming aware of the uncertainty which pervades professional judgement.

The impact of these developments in the technology and scope of medicine is widely felt within the profession—if less widely understood. Many doctors are involved daily in work for which their education and training has not prepared them—for example, handling potent interventions where the balance between risk and benefit is elusive. The considerable problems posed by uncertainty of this kind are compounded by changes in our society which have reshaped the context of practice; medical paternalism is no longer an acceptable basis for the doctor–patient relationship.

During the same period undergraduate medical education has changed only marginally from the process I experienced. Of course, scientific and technical advances feature in the curriculum and new subjects have been introduced, but the framework (including the duration) stands largely unmodified. Indeed, expansion of the knowledge base and the scope of medicine has made it even harder for medical students to integrate teaching from diverse sources, much of it poorly related to the actual tasks of clinical practice.

Postgraduate training is not designed to explore issues such as the scope of medicine but to impart a narrow range of diagnostic and therapeutic skills in the chosen specialty. It is only with the achievement of seniority and independence of action that doctors begin to recognise the inadequacies of their preparation for the role.

When confronted by patient's problems, doctors perceive doubts about their role centred on three questions: *Is there a problem?*; *Can I intervene safely and effectively?* and *Should others (within and outside medicine) be involved?* The wider role of doctors in relation to disease prevention and health promotion raises strikingly similar doubts. In this book David Seedhouse seeks to help doctors with these fundamental questions. He does so by reinstating uncertainty as a fact of professional life and by devising practical models to guide the clinician (and medical student) towards a realistic appraisal of the uncertainty implicit in medical intervention.

While all the ideas are not new, their application by Dr Seedhouse is both remarkably clear and immediately useful to doctors. The well-informed approach of the author is both sympathetic to and supportive of the role of the clinician; a refreshing change in non-medical writers about clinical practice. I venture to suggest that this will prove to be a seminal book, not least because it provides something we have long needed—a coherent strategy for undergraduate medical education.

Ian Stanley, MB, ChB, MRCS, MRCP, FRCGP
Professor of General Practice
University of Liverpool, UK

Preface

The best philosophy is helpful. Any worthwhile philosophical activity will encourage progress in either theory or practice, and sometimes in both. John Locke, a notable early eighteenth century philosopher, wrote in his *Essay Concerning Human Understanding*:

'The commonwealth of learning is not at this time without master builders . . . but everyone must not hope to be a Boyle or a Sydenham . . . it is ambition enough to be employed as an underlabourer in clearing the ground a little . . .'

This book sits firmly in this tradition, yet hopes to extend it. Philosophy is not only underlabouring, it is not only a process of clarification of meaning and theory. Philosophy can also construct, suggest and recommend as a result of thoughtful, logical analysis.

In this book the philosophical process is applied to three fundamental questions. These are: '*What is the purpose of medicine?*'; '*What is the medical doctor's legitimate role—in general and in specific circumstances?*'; and '*What are, and what ought to be, the limits on medical interventions?*'. These are daunting questions. Their answers are not easily found and cannot be given quickly. Yet these questions are central to an understanding of the medical endeavour. They are questions to which all medical practitioners should be able to offer considered responses.

This book is designed to assist doctors to arrive at an enhanced understanding of these vital issues. As such it is consistently positive. There are no idle fancies or abstractions to be found in this inquiry. Instead realistic answers are relentlessly and singlemindedly pursued. In the first two chapters Locke's 'underlabouring' is found to be necessary, but once the ground has been cleared of some common misperceptions a refreshing practical theory is constructed. Three beliefs are shovelled away: that medicine is a discipline which can and should always strive to move nearer to absolute certainty, that normality is a state which can be discovered without the addition of human judgement, and that disease is somehow a special category of human problem. These mistaken assumptions are replaced by a framework held firmly in place by a strong and workable theory of health, a practical tool to help doctors recognise clear limits to medical activity, and a simple 'litmus test' to help evaluate the moral status of any proposed intervention.

The purpose of this book is to *liberate medicine*. This, on the face of it might seem a strange task—not least because in recent years medical practice has been subject to a wide range of criticisms and proposals for reform. Usually it is the patient who is championed against a medical profession accused of wielding excessive power. Typically it is protested that medicine needs to be restrained in order to restrict its clinical enthusiasm and imperialism in health care. But it has never been suggested that medicine itself needs to be freed.

Medicine, as it is now, has not been designed but has evolved as a complex organism. As a result of this generally undirected development few have seriously addressed the question, '*Which direction* ought *medicine to take?*' From time to time some doctors ask: '*What is my proper role?*'; '*How far ought I to intervene in this person's life?*'; '*Where does my job end and another carer's responsibility start?*' or '*How far am I equipped to do good in this situation?*' From necessity such thoughtful doctors arrive at answers in specific cases, but even they find it far harder to reach firm conclusions about the general purpose of medicine. Part of the problem is that newly qualified doctors enter a profession which is so enormously complicated that they can only react to what exists. There is no time and, with little prospect of affecting change, apparently little point in their considering wholesale improvement.

Specifically medicine is currently constrained in the following unnecessary ways: by a clinical tradition which seriously overemphasises the extent to which certainty can be achieved in medical work; by an underdeveloped understanding of the many essential non-clinical aspects of medical work; and by the lack of a fully analysed rationale. Currently medicine does not possess a consistent philosophy of health.

Medical training equips a doctor with many technical skills, but few or no theoretical tools with which to examine the medical system itself. Nevertheless medicine needs direction. It is argued in this book that the best source of this orientation must be doctors themselves. Many clinicians feel that medicine is not achieving what it might, but are unable to articulate their feelings into comprehensive policies for growth. Doctors, searching for positive ways to progress, need the liberation which comes with clear sight.

The key to the liberation of medicine is for doctors to be helped to understand more clearly its theoretical drives. Through this heightened recognition of possible goals and potential limits doctors will be more free to select the most beneficial targets for their health work. As doctors become more able to plan their strategies for care freely within the limits to legitimate medical practice, so it becomes likely that they will be able to liberate more and broader fulfilling potentials in those for whom they seek to care.

Acknowledgements

Sadly Martha, Metz, Ulrig and the rest turned out to be a mirage. However, some certainties remain. Once again conversations with Alan Cribb and Harry Lesser proved invaluable. In particular Alan provided a vital impulse to my thinking about the Rings and the Autonomy Flip. Ian Stanley has constantly been extremely supportive during my time at Liverpool Medical School, and has taught me a great deal.

Much gratitude is due also to Karen Black who typed most of the manuscript, and kept me laughing. I cannot begin to thank Hilary enough.

Introduction

In order to assist growth in medicine* it has become essential to stand apart from a tradition of largely hostile external comment. This book seeks to analyse rather than condemn, to suggest rather than to prescribe, and to move on from a time when it was thought necessary to provoke change through conquest.

Medicine under Fire

Over the last two decades medicine has been roundly criticised from many quarters. Of the numerous assaults on medicine the two most famous critiques have been delivered by Ivan Illich [1] and Ian Kennedy [2]. Both writers launched telling attacks, but despite detailed research and argument, both polemics ultimately fail because they do not offer adequate theoretical foundations from which to construct *realistic proposals for progress*. In the absence of thoughtful alternatives to existing systems critiques tend to irritate rather than inspire.

These are Illich's main criticisms of medicine:

(1) Illich believes that medicine is a counter-productive enterprise, that medical intervention produces more harm than good. Illich accuses medicine of *iatrogenesis*—in other words he claims that doctors cause sickness. Illich lists extensive evidence of 'side-effects' of drugs actually worse than the problems they are prescribed to alleviate, and he cites equally detailed research of 'unnecessary surgery'.

(2) Illich argues that medicine reinforces political environments in which sickness and deviance can be defined only by those with medical authority. As a result doctors are in a position of tremendous influence and privilege. They, and only they, have the power to legitimise extended absence from work by defining a problem as an illness: doctors have the ultimate authority to declare which patient is mentally ill, which person is normal, and which deviant; and it is primarily in the hands of the doctor to say which child has been 'abused' and which child has not. Illich regards such decisions to be essentially political or social, not medical. He insists that by taking on a political role medicine has far outstepped its legitimate function.

(3) The most insidious product of medical activity is the weakening of the ability of individuals to cope, to heal themselves when ill, to change their environment, and to challenge the *status quo*. Illich believes that the deference of patients to doctors is now so exaggerated that they are scarcely able to deal with their own coughs or their baby's sneezes, without running to the 'medical man' for drugs and reassurance. He argues that many modern problems are caused by

---

*The word 'medicine' is normally used in this book to denote 'the discipline of medicine'.

environments which lead to stress, and which directly cause other illness. He asks, how will individuals begin to change their situations for themselves when they lack the confidence to deal with even minor problems?

Illich accuses doctors of fostering and being flattered by this dependency. He claims that medicine is undermining autonomy, and that the only way this most precious human asset can be restored is for lay people to say to medicine, 'Enough!' and begin to take control of their own destinies.

These are powerful criticisms, which Ian Kennedy reinforces.

Like Illich, Kennedy thinks that medicine has taken the wrong path. Unlike Illich, Kennedy thinks that medicine has been reasonably successful in the treatment of sickness; but as a result lay people have assumed that it is to medicine that they must turn to promote and maintain their health. However, for Kennedy 'being healthy' and 'not being ill' are not synonymous. He writes 'Health, if it is to have any useful meaning, must refer to more than the mere absence of illness'. But because the two ideas are popularly associated medicine has slowly taken on tasks for which it is not technically equipped. Medical training is essentially training in clinical science directed at identifying and treating disease, but because medical work is generally thought to be identical to health work many more decisions now fall under the remit of 'clinical judgement' than strictly ought to.

Kennedy argues that doctors frequently make decisions which are social, ethical, economic, and political in nature. Sometimes little—if any—of the content of these decisions is purely medical but—out of habit—all is assumed to fall under the umbrella of 'clinical judgement'.

Kennedy illustrates his case with many examples, including these.

(1) Who, asks Kennedy, decides who gets the kidney? When there are more patients who might benefit from a kidney transplant than there are available compatible kidneys, why does it fall to doctors to judge who will be lucky? Clinical considerations being equal, the decision is a moral, economic, and social one, so by what right is the allocation decision within the brief of doctors?

(2) Demand exceeds supply for fertility treatments such as *in vitro fertilisation* (IVF), *artificial insemination by donor* (DI), and *gamete fallopian tube transfer* (GIFT). Kennedy wonders why it should be that medics, with their particular sets of values, should draw up the waiting list for treatment. Almost invariably married couples are preferred before single-parents, lesbian couples or prostitutes. Clearly such value judgements—however much we approve or disapprove of them—have nothing to do with clinical practice. It is necessary for people with medical training to monitor the outcome of these procedures, but why should they have sole charge over the initial moral decision?

(3) On a related theme, Kennedy notes that in law the contraceptive pill must be given on prescription, but also that there is no medical consensus over the appropriate circumstances in which to offer it. For some groups of patients there can be a considerable element of lottery. Dependent upon her doctor's personal moral opinion a teenage girl may, or may not, receive the help she requires. Undeniably doctors are making value judgements in such cases. But, asks Kennedy, since contraception and pregnancy are not usually related

to disease, why are these taken to be legitimate matters for medical adjudication at all?

Kennedy believes that sexuality has nothing to do with medicine. If a person is sexually attracted to people of the same sex, that is her business, and not a matter for medicine. He uses this example to indicate that on occasions decisions about what are and are not diseases seem to be quite arbitrary. He quotes a decision taken by the American Psychiatric Association which voted in 1974 that homosexuality was not an illness. Before the vote homosexuality was a mental illness and afterwards it is not. Surely, argues Kennedy, questions about the nature and existence of disease should be based in science rather than in value.

Solutions?

Both Illich and Kennedy want changes to be made to medicine from the outside. They each demand that external forces impose new practices upon medicine.

Illich dreams of a near-utopia where the 'common man' is in control of his destiny. But this lack of realism is precisely his problem. He believes that the public should rise up to demand 'the demystification of all medical matters', and that the 'medical establishment' ought to be dismantled. He does not spell out how this is to happen, but he insists that the general populace must acquire the competence and confidence to evaluate the disastrous effects that medicine has had on public autonomy, and will then press for a fresh start. According to Illich people in Western society have been severely disabled by demands for workers to conform to the requirements of industry, by education for fixed roles and social positions, and by a 'medical establishment' which nourishes dependency. But given this, given the extent to which general human autonomy has supposedly been undermined, it is hard to imagine the mechanisms by which it is to be recovered solely through the efforts of an emasculated people.

Kennedy appears to take a more down-to-earth approach. He argues that since the majority of sickness is caused by deprivation of some kind, such as poverty of money or poverty of knowledge, resources should be directed away from the NHS towards the creation of a more equitable society: improvements in health must come through changes in the way people are able to live. He also argues that medicine should have a more carefully defined code of practice. This should be produced by 'a Permanent Standing Advisory Committee charged with the task of drawing up Codes of Practice and of keeping developments in medicine under constant review, with a view to identifying and responding to ethical issues'. The advisory committee would consist of specialists in medicine, ethics, law and economics, and would aim to produce, over time, a comprehensive Code of Practice governing the ethics of medical practice.

But the latter argument delivers Kennedy into a realm at least as fantastic as Illich's vision. If his suggestion is meant seriously it demonstrates a deep misunderstanding of both the nature of ethics and medical practice. The belief that it is possible to prescribe what is and is not ethical behaviour in medicine—where so much is uncertain and where a range of different opinions can each be valid alternatives—is simply wrong.

The problem with Kennedy's analysis is not that his conclusions are not worth considering, but that he has not thought through their basis sufficiently to be able to suggest to doctors ways in which they might choose to progress for themselves.

Not only does he give no convincing reasons why doctors should choose the ethical principles he espouses—respect for autonomy, truth-telling, promise keeping, respect for the dignity of the individual, and the principle of seeking to do justice—but *he does not say what health is*. And since he cannot say what health is all he can do is to criticise the present evolved goals of medical practice. Of course this is his primary purpose, but it leaves the reader both tantalised and exasperated. Kennedy's treatise owes more to deeply held opinion than developed philosophical argument. As a result he cannot derive revised targets for medicine from a solid theoretical base—his position allows him only enough rope to propose that many of the functions of medicine should be supervised by other professional groups. But to argue that external bodies impose new limits upon medicine is not only unrealistic, it is also ultimately negative. In effect it demeans doctors, it says to them 'you are unfit to be in sole control of your profession'. Not surprisingly many doctors have reacted angrily to what they perceive to be unnecessary aggression from a prejudiced outsider.

The question '*What's wrong with medicine?*' is considered in depth by both Illich and Kennedy. The questions '*What's medicine for?*', '*What role ought a doctor perform?*' and '*At what point should a doctor begin to intervene and when should he stop?*' are left untouched. The job is half-done.

Realism

Illich and Kennedy point to a negative side of medicine, and dream of radical change. Both claim that medicine is too powerful, and both suggest constraints. Neither of their visions of the future—medicine disempowered by popular pressure, and medicine shackled by committees of other professionals—are remotely plausible. Medicine is too large and complex an enterprise, and far too well-established, to bow to such enforced change—unless imposed by Statute.

As long as doctors continue to offer extensive human assistance in an uncertain world they must make judgements which are not strictly clinical. To decide whether or not to intervene in another person's life in a world of limited resources is, by its very nature, a social, economic and ethical judgement. Unless a doctor only ever deals with unconscious flesh, muscle, blood and bone, he must interact with people. And such interactions are always complex. Doctors must, of necessity, make general decisions in their professional capacities. At present most doctors are not well educated in such non-clinical skills, yet they are called upon to perform as if they are. Medical education produces doctors adept only at a range of specifically clinical subjects even though most will work as generalist health workers, as flexible carers who must make effective, sensitive decisions about both clinical and non-clinical issues.

It is time to liberate medicine from these paradoxes, and so to pave the way for a form of health care which is itself liberating. This book attempts to go beyond criticism to construction, in the knowledge that it is less difficult to say what is wrong than to state clearly how things might change for the better. The construction process builds on a broad theory of health, shows how the adoption of this theory will impose a number of limits on medical activity, and suggests ways of improving communication and understanding between health workers of all kinds.

The argument is likely to face criticism from those who believe that a great many social and health problems are caused and perpetuated by the very existence of a medical profession. Such a view is possibly partly correct, but is enormously difficult to establish with any certainty. It is also very hard to imagine developed societies, at least in the foreseeable future, which do not accord high status and power to those who work to heal through medicine.

However, the argument developed in this book is far from conservative. It is all the more radical for shunning explicit criticism of medicine and the existing political structures which maintain it. At its heart the book seeks to demonstrate that medicine might work for health in a way that welcomes care beyond the strictly clinical. At the same time it acknowledges that if the presence or absence of disease can no longer form the dividing line between legitimate and non-legitimate medical intervention, then alternative limits must be clarified. Without them doctors will have little guidance about where to begin and where to stop their work, and will be open to further accusations of 'medicalisation'. The aim of medicine, like all health care, should be to recognise and if possible to release optimum levels of human potential wherever this is feasible. This book suggests clear limits to medicine whilst arguing that within these limits doctors need liberating; they need new skills, and sometimes fresh attitudes, to move as freely and creatively as possible.

Part I

Uncertainty

Chapter One

What's the Problem?

Introduction

There is much in medicine that is certain*, but however far the clinician is able to extend the boundaries of certainty, he will, at some point, always step over into uncertainty. This chapter begins to illustrate this truth, which is the central theme of Part I.

Part I highlights uncertainty in medical activity. Although this topic is recognised in enlightened medical literature [3], it is not a traditional category of study and discussion in medical education. This is despite the fact that the work of doctors is essentially uncertain—that medicine without uncertainty is like history without the past. Much medical education instils the belief that the clinician's role is to probe until he has finally uncovered certainty. The reason why doctors take histories, for instance, is not to float possible answers for quiet discussion, but to get to the tap-root of a problem as soon as possible. Either a person has cancer of the rectum or he does not. It is the clinical scientist's job to discover the truth about disease, and then to suggest the best treatment. The message is that uncertainty changes to certainty given the proper application of medical skill; the role of medicine is to beat uncertainty not to accommodate it.

There are several types and levels of uncertainty in medicine. It is essential that multiple technical skills are transmitted to doctors in order to enable them to cope with clinical and therapeutic ambiguities—and to encourage the best possible medical solutions. But it is equally necessary that multiple non-clinical abilities are developed in doctors in order to facilitate strategies to tackle the diverse uncertainties generated by caring for other people.

A possible case of anorexia nervosa is offered as an initial illustration of multiple uncertainty in medicine. No-one knows what causes anorexia nervosa. And although the condition is currently classed as a disease, and some people die as a result of self-starvation, no-one can be sure of the best treatment for anorexia. Add to this picture doubt about the ethics of forcible intervention in the life of 'an anorexic', the possibility of substantial misperception about the aims of 'the sufferer', and the emotional pain which attends the desire to help someone who is deliberately not eating, then a sea of uncertainty comes into view.

Anorexia is generally acknowledged to be difficult for medicine to categorise and to deal with, but it is not an exceptional case. Uncertainty pervades medicine, and the challenge of dealing with it in its various manifestations is part of the

---

*Or at least as close to certainty as can be in an imperfect world.

3

attraction of the profession. Even when the tumour has been detected with certainty the prognoses of people who have cancer remains uncertain. The results of surgical operations can be predicted only up to a degree of probability since each operation and patient is unique. Statistical analysis can predict trends and probabilities, but is unable to provide absolute certainty. Statistically, the chance of success of a particular operation to relieve pressure on a nerve root is approximately 98%, but which patients will fall into the category of the unfortunate 2% and be injured is not predictable [4].

Whenever medicine achieves certainty in one aspect of care the only other certainty is that there is further uncertainty ahead. Once schizophrenia is diagnosed it is difficult—if not impossible—to predict whether the patient will have only a single psychotic episode, will have repeated episodes with remissions, or will degenerate chronically. A diagnosis of multiple sclerosis can mean that a person will become blind and paralysed within 10 years, if not sooner, or it can mean that a person can live her life untroubled by anything more than occasional 'pins and needles'.

A doctor cannot help but face uncertainty. How she deals with it is a reflection both of her competence and her humanity.

Struggling with Uncertainty

Imagine this scenario.

Michael Clarke, a young doctor, recently qualified as a principal in general practice, is sitting awaiting his next patient at a regular morning surgery. He calls up the records of Shirley Brown on his computer screen, and wonders idly what the 17-year-old might want of him. Her history shows nothing remarkable.

There is a brisk knock and Shirley's mother walks in, holding Shirley by the hand. Dr Clarke turns away from the records to greet his visitors. He had retained an image of Shirley from her last visit when she was concerned about a throat infection. Nine months ago he thought she was highly attractive. She was obviously intelligent and articulate, and about to begin college to take A-levels. But now she is dramatically changed.

Dr Clarke normally sets aside approximately eight minutes to deal with each patient, but immediately decides that he must abandon this rule for the mother and daughter. He can see that both have been crying, but Shirley looks truly dreadful. Her face is so thin that the contours of her skull are striking. Her yellow hair is tied back, drawn away from her face, so that the shock is heightened. She is wearing a black pleated skirt down to her knees, and shoes with heels that tense her calf muscles, giving the impression that the covering skin is almost transparent.

Shirley's mother begins to speak, rapidly explaining that she is terrified that Shirley will die because she just will not eat. She pleads that she has reached the point where she cannot cope with her daughter without help. While her mother is speaking Shirley sits, seemingly impassive, staring into the middle distance. After listening to the mother—and observing Shirley—Dr Clarke judges that it is best to speak to Shirley alone. He explains this, upon which her mother agrees to wait outside, and to speak to him after he has seen Shirley in private.

Dr Clarke speaks softly to Shirley: "I'm sorry you are so upset Shirley, what's the problem?"

Shirley replies assertively, "I don't have a problem. Mum wants me to eat when I don't want to. I'm not hungry so I don't eat—it's simple."

"Well, you are much thinner than you were the last time I saw you. Do you have any pains?"

"No, I'm fine."

"Have you been feeling tired . . . lethargic?"

"No, not at all. I'm just my normal self."

"Have you been having normal periods?"

"Um . . . I don't have heavy periods at all."

"When was your last period?"

Shirley hesitates, then replies, "About four months ago, but I'm definitely not pregnant!"

"Have you been depressed . . . unhappy?"

"I'm happy at college, when I'm working. I love to work. It's better when I'm left alone."

After a brief monologue on his similar study habits as a medical student, Dr Clarke returns the conversation to the subject of food.

"What did you eat for breakfast today?"

"Tomato juice".

"Is that all?"

"I'm not hungry in the morning. What do you eat for breakfast?"

"Toast usually, then sandwiches for lunch, and a main meal in the evening. What's a typical main meal for you?"

"I like salad, especially now that it's summer. I must watch my weight."

Dr Clarke takes the opportunity to focus on Shirley's weight.

"Shirley, would you object to being weighed now?"

"There's no point. I can tell you. I weighed myself this morning. I'm 6 st 2 lbs."

"Have you ever been this low before, I mean apart from when you were a child?"

"I've been far too fat before."

"Judith, that's your older sister isn't it, has she ever worried your mother in this way?"

"I haven't deliberately worried Mum. I don't want to hurt her. I wish that she would not get at me all the time about eating."

"What does your father think about this?"

"He's away a lot on business. He shouts at me at the table sometimes—he says I'm picking, but it's when I've had enough to eat."

Dr Clarke pauses and considers. Shirley is adamantly resisting his attempts to have her admit that she has a problem, and he needs to find out more. He asks her, "Shirley, would you mind if I talk to your mother for a little while, on our own? Would you wait on the chair just outside? I'll ask the receptionist to make sure that you are not disturbed."

Shirley leaves, and her mother, Angela, enters the consulting room. She is still distressed, but sits down to talk to Dr Clarke, who attempts to take a more detailed history. He inquires about when and what Shirley eats. He asks when it was that Angela first noticed the weight loss, whether anything similar has happened before, whether Shirley has ever had a psychological problem—perhaps a phobia? And then—carefully—he inquires how the family is getting on. How's Judith? How's Shirley getting on at college? Are there any problems at home? Are there any tensions? Angela replies that she noticed about nine months ago that Shirley was off her food, and about six months ago she was really very thin, but about a stone heavier than now. Other than this she thinks that she can be little help to him—she is at a loss to explain what is happening, and is very frightened by it. Whatever she tries, Shirley won't eat. She hardly sees her eat anything. Judith is great—she's getting on well as a secretary at an insurance broker's, and has a steady boyfriend. Shirley's college work is good; in fact she seems obsessed by it, she's working harder and longer than ever. Life at home was settled, perfectly normal, until Shirley developed this problem.

Dr Clarke decides that he needs time to think. He has already formed and tested some general hypotheses. He has considered that there might be a physical cause for the weight loss—but has not yet detected any plausible possibilities. It seems more likely that the problem is psychological. He has ruled out depression because Shirley is working so energetically. And as she seems quite in touch with reality she is unlikely to be suffering from a psychotic illness. He strongly suspects that Shirley is a victim of anorexia nervosa, although he has never encountered a person with the disease before. Since Shirley's weight loss does not seem to be totally out of control he believes she is not in immediate physical danger. He calls Shirley in and asks Angela and her to return in three days.

Michael Clarke remembers Shirley, rather fondly, as one of his first patients. He is satisfied that although he is not yet sure of its nature Shirley definitely has a problem. He is so concerned by the dramatic change in her that he decides he must take a special interest in her case.

In taking the decision to step in he has answered the first part of a central question for any doctor: 'Should I intervene, and if so, how?' Before he addresses the second part of the question Dr Clarke cautiously resolves to confirm his suspicion, and then to seek the views of his more experienced colleagues about how best to proceed.

First Uncertainties

It is at this point that Dr Clarke confronts the first uncertainties. On checking, he is surprised to find that the diagnostic criteria for anorexia nervosa are not clear-cut. He discovers three alternative sets [5]. Dr Clarke must decide which is correct, but is unsure how to judge between them.

Alternatives

On scanning each set of criteria (Tables 1.1–1.3) Dr Clarke notices that there appears to be a progressive slackening of the conditions necessary for a diagnosis of anorexia. During his reading after surgery he discovers yet another set of criteria [6], but he decides that he must restrict his dilemma to choosing between the three most

Table 1.1 Feighner criteria for anorexia nervosa

a. Age of onset prior to 25.
b. Anorexia with accompanying weight loss of at least 25% of original body weight.
c. A distorted, implacable attitude toward eating, food, or weight that overrides hunger, admonitions, reassurance and threats, e.g.
    (1) denial of illness with a failure to recognise nutritional needs;
    (2) apparent enjoyment in losing weight, with overt manifestation that food refusal is a pleasurable indulgence;
    (3) a desired body image of extreme thinness, with overt evidence that it is rewarding to the patient to achieve and maintain this state; and
    (4) unusual hoarding or handling of food.
d. No known medical illness that could account for the anorexia and weight loss.
e. No other known psychiatric disorder with particular reference to primary affective disorder, schizophrenia, and obsessive-compulsive and phobic neurosis. (The assumption is made that even though it may appear phobic or obsessional, food refusal alone is not sufficient to qualify for obsessive-compulsive or phobic disease).

For a diagnosis of anorexia nervosa, 'a' through to 'e' are required and

f. At least two of the following manifestations:
    (1) amenorrhoea (no menstruation)
    (2) lanugo (fine body hair)
    (3) bradycardia (persistent resting pulse of 60 or less)
    (4) periods of overactivity
    (5) episodes of bulimia (bingeing on food), or
    (6) vomiting which may be self-induced.

Table 1.2 DSM-III* diagnostic criteria for anorexia nervosa

a. Intense fear of becoming obese, which does not diminish as weight loss progresses.
b. Disturbance of body image, e.g. claiming to 'feel fat' even when emaciated.
c. Weight loss of at least 25% of original body weight; or if under 18 years of age, weight lost from original body weight plus projected weight gain expected from growth charts may be combined to make 25%.
d. Refusal to maintain body weight over a minimal normal weight for age and height.
e. No known physical illness that would account for the weight loss.

*DSM-III refers to the American Psychiatric Association's 'Diagnostic and Statistical Manual of Mental Disorders', 3rd edition, 1980.

Table 1.3 DSM-III-R criteria for anorexia nervosa

a. Refusal to maintain body weight for age and height and which results in maintenance of body weight 15% below expected; failure to make expected weight gain for the growth period which also results in maintenance of body weight 15% below expected for height and age.
b. Intense fear of becoming overweight, even when underweight.
c. Body-image disturbance—claiming to 'feel fat' even when emaciated (this usually takes the form of the patient believing parts of the body, hips for example, are fat when they are in fact obviously underweight).
d. In females, the absence of at least three consecutive menstrual cycles when otherwise expected to occur—primary or secondary amenorrhoea.

commonly referenced. On surveying the options in more detail he notes that the DSM-III criteria are distinctly less precise than the Feighner diagnostic standard. On DSM-III there is no age limit, and few specific behaviours or attitudes are required for a diagnosis. The proposed DSM-III-R criteria are more flexible still. It is 'the intense fear of becoming overweight' that is stressed, and a loss of only 15% of expected body weight for height is required for a diagnosis. This is significantly less than the 25% necessary on the other sets of criteria. In concrete terms, 15% of 8 st 7 lbs is 18 lbs. So, in order to satisfy criterion (a) on the DSM-III-R scale, a young woman who would be expected to weigh 8 st 7 lbs must weigh 7 st 3 lbs or less—which is by no means unequivocally abnormal.

Dr Clarke has begun to tread a little further into uncertainty. His first dilemma was 'does Shirley have a problem or does her mother merely think she has a problem?' However, having come to a judgement on this question, he now has to choose which diagnostic criteria to use. Unfortunately for Dr Clarke there is no single authoritative opinion to guide him in this decision.

Although he does not yet appreciate it Dr Clarke is attempting to come to grips with an uncertainty which saturates medicine. He is aware that he will have to make at least one partially subjective judgement when he decides which set of criteria to use. In addition, he recognises that the DSM-III-R test seems to qualify many other women as anorexic who would not think of themselves as ill. He knows that at some point many girls and women (and some men) choose to lose substantial amounts of weight. Simple observation shows that in most Western societies there is a strong cultural tendency, especially for women, to watch their weight and to worry if they put on more than a few pounds. And Dr Clarke's clinical experience has taught him that it is not uncommon for women to report menstrual irregularity of two to three cycles, especially if they are stressed. However, the basic underlying issue is: *What is normal?* In order to help Shirley sooner or later Dr Clarke must address this question, if only implicitly.

But Michael Clarke does not have the time to think about the general problem of normality at the moment. His urgent concern is Shirley. She is 5 ft 7 ins tall and, at 17 years old, ought to weigh between 8 st 7 lbs and 9 st 7 lbs. Her present weight of 6 st 2 lbs is approximately 27% less than the lowest weight she might be expected to be. Thus her weight qualifies her as anorexic on all three sets of diagnostic criteria.

Dr Clarke resolves to arrive at a firm diagnosis at the next consultation. He does not want to make a mistake with Shirley, defining her as ill if she is well. So, in order to ensure that he does not do her any injustice, he decides to work with the Fieghner criteria to arrive at his final diagnosis. He is not certain that these are the correct set to use, but they do seem to be the most thorough, and so the safest and best guide. He sets aside time at the end of his Thursday surgery to see Shirley and her mother. He sees them both together and attempts to check the various Feighner conditions. On questioning, and on astute listening to the points on which they disagree, he reaches some provisional conclusions.

A diagnosis

Shirley has abnormal eating patterns. There can be little doubt about this, and there is no question that Shirley appears to enjoy her extreme thinness. Dr Clarke can find no physical reason for her weight loss, other than that Shirley is not eating enough food. Shirley has no history of psychiatric disorder, neither has the family reported mental illness in the past. Her excessive attention to her college work is patently over-enthusiastic, but it does not appear to be a manifestation of a deeper psychiatric difficulty. Shirley is not anxious about failure, or concerned to keep up with her peer group. It seems that she works as hard as she does because it pleases her, and this is not usually indicative of mental illness. Dr Clarke muses that if working extremely hard in order to achieve a desired goal is a sign of mental illness then many medical students, business people, and athletes are in need of psychiatric help.

Dr Clarke is unable to ascertain conclusively whether or not there have been episodes of bulimia ('bingeing' large quantities of food) or vomiting. Shirley does not have lanugo, but since this is naturally associated with very low weight, he does not consider its presence or absence to be of much significance. However, he has been able to establish that she is often extremely active, has missed four menstrual cycles (amenorrhoea) and that her pulse is persistently less than 60 beats per minute (bradycardia).

After seeming to move backwards by encountering uncertainty about the diagnostic measures, Dr Clarke now appears to have advanced. He feels that he may have pushed the boundary separating certainty from uncertainty further away from him. *If the Feighner criteria accurately define anorexia nervosa, then Shirley has the disease.* However, Dr Clarke is acutely aware of the hypothetical nature of this statement. He remains unsure of the legitimacy of the criteria, but he feels he must make some decisions. He cannot be paralysed by scepticism, however well founded it is.

At least now his problem has changed. Now he has to decide what, if anything, further to do about Shirley's anorexia nervosa. In order to begin to deal with this next uncertainty he turns to his more experienced colleagues.

On chatting to the three medical colleagues who share his practice Michael receives three different opinions, all of which conflict at some point. He knows that this is not unusual [7, 8], but it complicates rather than simplifies matters. It impedes his effort to push the dividing line between certainty and uncertainty further from him.

Possible therapies

Dr Clarke is worried, although not only for Shirley. He is anxious about doing the best for all concerned in a difficult situation, and he naturally wants to be seen to succeed. He knows that he might attempt to deal with the problem single-handed at least initially, and he knows that he could refer Shirley on. There are risks for Shirley associated with either option, and there are associated risks for him. If he takes responsibility for Shirley, and her condition worsens, then he will feel that he has failed. If he refers her, and she improves with treatment, then he may ponder that he might have succeeded himself. And if she were to deteriorate on referral, then he would be open to the accusation of having made the wrong choice. Should Dr Clarke take on a role where he assumes sole responsibility for Shirley? Should he share the work with others, or should he pass her on entirely? Crucially, how is the doctor to judge where his appropriate role begins and ends? How can he decide upon the limits to his usefulness as a medical doctor?

Dr Clarke attempts to confront these questions. He first seeks the opinion of his senior partner, who tells him that he ought to try to deal with the situation himself. Since he has singled Shirley out for special attention he ought to commit the necessary time to her. The senior partner suggests that Dr Clarke should take a consistently firm line with the patient as far as her eating habits are concerned, and that he should be prepared to remove the responsibility of overseeing her performance from her mother. He should allow her to talk about her feelings and her problems, he should weigh her every week, and he should reward weight gain. The senior partner also reminds Dr Clarke of the mortality rate from anorexia, which he says is 5%—in other words there is a 1 in 20 chance that Shirley will die as a result of her disease.

On being reminded of this information Dr Clarke begins to feel threatened. It is one thing to rise to the intellectual challenge of 'hitting the right diagnosis', yet quite another to confront the fact that to make a bad choice means Shirley might die when she could have been helped to live. Fleetingly he is conscious of a vivid image from his postgraduate training:

$$\text{Perceived threat} = \frac{\text{Need for action}}{\text{Diagnostic certainty}}$$

Moving this thought to the forefront of his mind, Dr Clarke hurries to discuss the case, over coffee, with the remaining two partners. He begins by reporting the opinion of the senior partner, but Dr Smith is quick to interrupt. He argues that it boils down to a question of resources, and a busy general practitioner simply does not have the time to devote to such a complex problem. Dr Smith suggests to Dr Clarke that he must be realistic about the amount of time required for individual counselling, work with the family, and prolonged attention to Shirley's eating patterns. What about Dr Clarke's other patients? Are their needs less important? Hasn't Shirley caused some of this problem herself? Shirley should be referred for specialist help forthwith. Dr Smith highly recommends Dr Lawrence, a local consultant psychiatrist, and briefly describes the specialist's approach.

If Shirley were to be referred to Dr Lawrence he would probably first try to make a 'contract' with Shirley as an out-patient. The psychiatrist would seek to seal an agreement that if she was able to reach a set weight by a set date then her admission to hospital might be avoided. However, if the target could not be met—if the contract were to be broken—then Shirley would be admitted to the local psychiatric hospital, where she would remain until she had reached an 'ideal' or 'target' weight. This would probably be at least 8 st 7 lb in Shirley's case. The therapy used would be behaviour modification. In other words the treatment would be based on a system of reward for 'good behaviour' and punishment for 'bad behaviour'.

At 6 st 2 lbs Dr Smith thinks it unlikely that Dr Lawrence would allow the patient out of bed until she had gained at least one and a half stones. Shirley would be placed on a high-calorie diet in order to restore her weight as quickly as possible, and she would not be allowed a choice about what to eat. Drug treatment would probably be necessary, especially at first. In order to lessen tension and agitation chlorpromazine or other sedative phenothiazine might be used in large doses. Later, as weight is regained, psychotherapeutic discussions, involving the family whenever appropriate, would be introduced. Any privileges, such as watching television, having books to read, and having people to talk to, would be offered gradually as weight is gained. Dr Smith recognises that this might sound tough on the girl but the crucial factor in all this is that she must put on weight—once this is sorted out then her other problems can be tackled.

Dr Green, who has been listening with growing impatience to Dr Smith, disagrees forcibly. She insists that this standard psychiatric approach is likely to be counterproductive and woefully misunderstands the nature of anorexia. Dr Green curtly refers Dr Clarke to the feminist literature on anorexia nervosa. She explains that, in her opinion, anorexic women suffer deep internal conflicts, and often feel that life is out of control. An anorexic woman feels tossed by external forces and pressures. As a last resort she will turn inwards to find something that she can control, discovering that what she puts into her mouth is up to her and no-one else. By limiting food intake she is asserting her independence in the only area of her existence she can. In effect she is rejecting 'the outside' which she feels is in control of her. She is spurning all foreign substances and subjecting them to her will. Food comes to represent the alien outside forces—but she has come to be in command of food.

Dr Green insists that for a hospital to force Shirley to eat would be to take away the last vestige of control she has over her life—apart from suicide. Such a policy would drag her from the safety of her fragile world—a world in which she has finally become powerful—and subject her instead to a system of reward and punishment which might work reasonably well with rats, but which is quite inappropriate with people.

An approach to treatment which focuses solely on weight gain will make her feel even more of a failure than she does already. She will see her new 'fat' body as a sign of her weakness at giving in to the pressures of her family, the doctors and nurses to eat.

Dr Green insists that what is lowest in anorexic women is not weight but self-esteem. An anorexic girl has very little confidence, and it ought to be the task of a proper medical service to enable her to begin to take more charge of her life. Dr Clarke should be helping her to rebuild. He should resist the simplistic view that the restoration of Shirley's weight is the magic key to the resurrection of her life.

For Dr Green the real answer is to begin with Shirley, to start with what she would like to do with her life, not what she does or does not want to have for dinner. If Shirley agrees then she should be referred to a counsellor experienced in a range of methods, including psychotherapy, who has knowledge of the problems faced by anorexics. If Shirley does not agree that she needs treatment, if after conversations with Dr Clarke or the therapist she does not say 'yes, I would like help', then she should be left alone; there is no justification for interfering with her unless her life is in danger *and* she says that she does not want to die. Dr Clarke should not insist on 'refeeding' because this is a battleground of anorexia, not a seedbed for personal regrowth. Dr Green believes that the refeeding regime fuels a basic instinct to resist which is universally strong in anorexics. However, she does agree that Shirley should be encouraged to eat more if at all possible.

All Dr Clarke's colleagues agree that Shirley must put on weight, but do not concur about how Shirley is to be helped to achieve this goal.

In the face of this array of opinion, how is Dr Clarke to decide what to do? Should he do anything? Where can he find the scientific evidence to decide between the alternative suggestions? Where is the objective test? He seems almost to be drowning in questions, and he has to face the fact that there is no perfect method for arriving at *the* solution. He recognises that he will have to depend upon a personal judgement taken in the light of the available evidence—such as it is.

Although it can be said that some anorexics die, some make a partial recovery, and some return to 'normal' weight, even this 'evidence' is disputed. Experts disagree about the numbers which fall into each category, what counts as 'partial' and 'full' recovery is open to interpretation, and not all people become anorexic as a result of the sorts of difficulties Shirley is experiencing. Since people are complex and live unique lives the therapy which appears to have worked for one patient might not work—or may even prove disastrous—for another.

Crossing into Deeper Uncertainty

Deeper uncertainty—uncertainty more fundamental than puzzles about facts—awaits Dr Clarke. This uncertainty arises inevitably out of the desire of one person to intervene in the life of another. To intervene in another person's life, in whatever circumstances—whether by request or not—can have profound implications for either or both parties. This may be true of even apparently minor interventions. Telling a 'white lie', listening when a person needs to talk, offering constructive criticism, being arrogant or disdainful, can sometimes have far-reaching repercussions. It is well known that the effect we have when we touch other people's lives is never fully predictable, or detectable. This *uncertainty effect* is often most volatile in the case of interventions made by medical doctors.

Four basic questions which highlight further uncertainty

As Dr Clarke is making a decision about whether and how to intervene (and if he prefers the advice of Dr Green he might decide to call a halt to his intervention, even though a disease has been diagnosed), uncertainties beyond those of diagnosis, treatment and outcome come into play. These uncertainties can be highlighted by asking four simple questions.

The following simple questions might be asked by any doctor as soon as a patient presents for help. However, it will be shown later in this book, that the emphasis on illness is not as appropriate as it might first appear. Consequently, once it has been established that a problem exists, Dr Clarke's original key question '*Should I intervene, and if so how?*' is to be preferred as the opening question. However, raising these simple questions serves to demonstrate the presence of further uncertainty for the doctor.

The questions are:

(1) Is Shirley (or the patient in question) ill?
(2) If Shirley is ill, in what sense is she ill?
(3) Does her illness impair her reasoning ability to such an extent that she is incapable of making a cogent decision?
(4) How can the best solution to the problem be found for Shirley, taking into account the wellbeing of other people who might be affected?

All these questions can be subsumed under the central question, '*Should I intervene, and if so how?*' This question needs to be asked continually, even while the other questions are being asked, until it is concluded that no further intervention should be made. For example, if the answer to the question '*Is Shirley ill?*' is 'No', then there can be no professional justification for a medical intervention where medicine is conceived of as 'anti-disease' or 'anti-illness' work (unless Shirley says that she wishes to be helped to avoid potential illness, or unless there is some State policy or legal duty for professionals to enforce 'disease-avoiding behaviours). Since disease and illness is the traditional subject of medical work, where it is not present then it is difficult, at this stage in the analysis, to see how medicine might have a legitimate role.

If the answer to the question '*Is Shirley ill?*' is 'Yes' (as Dr Clarke judges), and if the answer to the second question '*In what sense is Shirley ill?*' is 'Shirley has a physical illness which is not affecting her thinking', then the justification for medical intervention becomes a little stronger, but only if the girl requests medical assistance. If Shirley is considered to be suffering solely from a physical illness, and does not want treatment, then her situation can be paralleled with that of a man who has a bleeding peptic ulcer, who has been taken by friends to the casualty department of the nearest hospital, but who chooses to refuse treatment. In such a case there is nothing that a doctor can do with legal, or more arguably, moral justification to prevent him bleeding to death. If there is no suggestion that the physical injury has caused impairment to his mental functioning, then there is a very strong case that he should be left alone.

Ethical uncertainty: *Should I intervene?*

Whenever anyone intervenes in the life of another person ethical issues will arise. In some interventions these issues are more obvious than in others. What if the answer to the first question—'*Is Shirley ill?*'—is 'No', although Dr Clarke is of the strong opinion that none the less, whether she thinks so or not, Shirley needs help. What if Shirley is only 14% below her expected body weight, but she and her family seem to be in a terrible emotional mess? Or what if Dr Clarke decides that anorexia nervosa is too nebulous an idea to count as an illness? Must Dr Clarke accept the argument that the family's distress is none of his concern? Such an argument might run like this.

If Shirley Brown wants to be very thin, and if her dieting is causing distress to her family, this is sad for her parents, but it is nothing more than a 'fact of life'. Inevitably children upset their parents. If doctors intervened every time a son worried his father they would have no time to treat genuinely sick people. The family should be left alone. Distress is a part of life. It may be that it is only through suffering that happiness means anything.

Why pick on Shirley, when she has a friend called Peter, whose father weighs 20 st, drinks heavily, smokes and takes no exercise. Even though Peter's father weighs over 33% of the expected normal weight for a man of 42, 5 ft 8 ins tall, he is not in danger of being treated against his will. Peter's father has taken clear risks in terms of disease, and he knows it. But still he chooses to continue to gamble with his life. Yet medicine does not suggest that he is ill, only that he is likely to become so if he carries on with his 'unhealthy' habits.

This is essentially the argument advanced by the man with the peptic ulcer who wishes to bleed to death. Would this argument completely tie Dr Clarke's hands, or might he follow a different line? Might Dr Clarke adopt the view that as a doctor of medicine, as a practical man, he cannot afford to spend too much time debating questions of meaning—but must act as soon as possible? Whether Shirley is actually ill or not, she is underweight and malnourished, and she is part of an emotionally disturbed family. If she does not already have a medically recognised illness she soon will have unless something is done for her. And even if she never crosses the border into a diseased state she and her family nevertheless have a problem which could be solved with appropriate care. Such an argument might make an appeal to the doctor's duty to 'resolve suffering', or might refer to the potentially dire consequences of letting the matter ride.

Which 'ethical approach' should Dr Clarke take? His difficulty is that he is a reasonable man. He can see the point of both arguments, and he is deeply unsure about what to do. He wonders if the law might help, as it has helped him in the past, when he took the decision to permit an abortion.

Legal uncertainty: *Should I invoke the law?*

If it is felt that the following answers to questions (1), (2), (3) and (4) are appropriate, then a different type of intervention becomes a possibility.

(1)   Yes, Shirley is ill.
(2)   Shirley has a mental illness. (These answers are implicit in the decision to describe Shirley's condition as anorexia nervosa.)
(3)   This illness has impaired her reasoning ability. (This is arguable in the case of anorexia nervosa.)
(4)   Her family want her to be treated even though she does not.

The case for a more forthright intervention becomes stronger still if it is clear that there is a risk of death.

If Dr Clarke does decide to intervene further in Shirley's life he has the option of reinforcing his medical practice by recourse to law. Specifically, he might use a Section of the Mental Health Act 1983. Shirley's mother and father can apply to have their daughter admitted for treatment in hospital under Section 3 of the Act, provided two doctors (one of whom must have substantial experience of psychiatry) give supporting written recommendations. In one respect delegation to law might allow Dr Clarke to feel that he has pushed the limits of his uncertainty out to the very end of his outstretched arms. By resorting to the law Dr Clarke might hope to alleviate both his anxiety and responsibility by deferring to statutory authority. Section 3 of the Mental Health Act makes it possible to place a person in hospital compulsorily for her own good or for the protection of other people.

Mental Health Act 1983 (Section 3)—admission for treatment

'This Section provides for the admission of a patient to hospital and his detention for treatment for a maximum period of six months (unless the order is renewed). The application may be made by the nearest relative or an approved social worker, founded upon the written recommendations of two doctors (one 'approved') who must indicate the, grounds for their opinion and why other methods of dealing with the patient are inappropriate. The grounds which may support an application are (a) that the patient is suffering from mental illness, severe mental impairment, psychopathic disorder or mental impairment and his mental disorder is of a nature or degree which makes it appropriate for him to receive medical treatment in hospital; and (b) in the case of psychopathic disorder or mental impairment, such treatment is likely to alleviate or prevent a deterioration of his condition; and (c) it is necessary for the health or safety of the patient or for the protection of other persons that he should receive such treatment and it cannot be provided unless he is detained under this Section. The patient has a right to apply to a Mental Health Review Tribunal within the first six months and once during each subsequent period for which the detention is renewed.' [9]

If it is judged that Shirley has an incapacitating mental illness, it becomes a legitimate option to detain her under Section 3. But although this may be a possible solution, and although it may turn out that Shirley is helped by it, eliciting the support of law gives only the impression that uncertainty has been eradicated. Uncertainty may be submerged but the question of whether or not to treat another person forcibly persists as a huge ethical issue.

Although the 1983 Mental Health Act is fairly clear about the conditions which must be met if a person is to be detained there are nevertheless legal uncertainties in mental health care. Once doctors have defined mental illness, and the other two conditions under Section Three are also satisfied, then treatment can legally go ahead without the consent of the patient. However, such treatment as is undertaken must still be carried out with reasonable care. To fall below this standard is to become open to an accusation of negligence [10]. For instance, if Shirley were to become emotionally damaged as the result of inept psychotherapy sessions, and causation could be established, then she might well sue the psychotherapist for negligence. To give another example, the law relating to sterilisation and abortion operations on patients defined as mentally incompetent is presently in the process of development, and must be described at least as being open to interpretation [11].

In addition to 'basic' *ethical and legal uncertainty* there are two other types which can usefully be distinguished at this stage. Since he cares, whatever he decides to do for Shirley, Dr Clarke must encounter these uncertainties. They might be called *uncertainty of interpretation* and *uncertainty of self*.

Uncertainty of interpretation: *Do I have this problem in the right context? Am I using the correct categories in my reasoning?*

Uncertainty of interpretation can stem either from the wide changes of emphasis which occur across different historical periods, societies, and cultures, or arise out of difficulty in the perceptions of individual people. Interpretations of health, disease, and even what are considered to be problems can change dependent upon time, place, and who is making the judgement. Once people now said to have psychiatric problems were said to be evil—possessed by devils [12]; a life expectancy of 45 years was accepted as the norm [13]; and a well-rounded female body was held to be the ideal [14]. But now the interpretation of such circumstances has changed.

In some situations Shirley's condition might not be interpreted as a problem. Even in our present culture it is generally felt to be appropriate for certain groups of young people, for instance jockeys or ballerinas, to reduce their weight intentionally to levels that, if it were not for their working status, would fall within the classification of anorexia. It is well known that highly trained women athletes are prone to amenorrhoea, but for non-professionals it is likely that the condition would be taken to be an indicator of disease.

One uncertainty of interpretation is in part also an uncertainty of self. This uncertainty rests in the possibility that the doctor might be misinterpreting the patient's symptoms, emotions or intentions, and that this might itself be creating a problem. Dr Clarke would like to understand Shirley's situation as clearly as possible. What is Shirley trying to do? Is what is happening to her quite out of her control, as if her trouble were influenza, or is she generating a necessary stage in her development as a woman—a stage in which medical interference is unwarranted and likely to be undermining or diminishing? Just as people choose to make sacrifices in their social life to become top-class athletes or academics, is Shirley choosing to be excessively thin as a means to a greater end? How can her past and present life be properly interpreted by a clinician armed only with 'common sense' and technical skills? How can Dr Clarke gain access to the truth as it is for Shirley?

Uncertainty of Self: *How is this going to affect me?*

This uncertainty primarily concerns the psychology of the individual carer. There is a tendency in some contemporary writings on health care ethics and politics to stress the rights and feelings of the person being cared for to a greater degree than those of the health worker. But the carer should be of equal concern in an analysis designed to develop the most creative response to any situation. Carers should not be thought of as impervious to the stresses of caring, or worse, as sacrificial objects.

The doctor can be vulnerable, unsure and selfish—he does not work as a neutral colourless machine, but as a person. Dr Clarke, for instance, is not a general practitioner purely for financial reward. He works for other benefits too [15], and when these are threatened then his security in what he is doing is threatened also.

A major reward for Dr Clarke, derived from his privileged position as a general practitioner, is that he is able to form special, trusting relationships with many of his patients. When a special relationship becomes strained it begins to become devalued. Truthfulness is a prerequisite for a trusting relationship, and on meeting her again Dr Clarke has recognised that even if she is not yet lying outright, Shirley is deliberately keeping information from him. She will not admit to vomiting or bulimia even though it is highly likely that these conditions are present, and she has attempted to conceal her amenorrhoea. Dr Clarke suspects that Shirley doesn't trust him to do what she wants—that she doesn't consider him to be her agent, but to be a potential antagonist.

As he deliberates about what his next intervention ought to be Dr Clarke confronts a further risk to himself—he grows increasingly uneasy about his emotions and motives. As he talks to Shirley for the second time in three days he begins to feel anger towards her. Although he is devoting a considerable amount of time to her she seems to be rejecting him in inverse proportion to his concern for her. Despite his genuine effort she will not relate to him, and he worries hard about the motives which lay beneath his developing preference to refer her to Dr Lawrence, the psychiatrist. Is he moving towards this conclusion because it is the best clinical option, or out of a sense of injustice—out of a feeling that Shirley is being unfair to him? Does he want to send her for behavioural and drug therapy as a punishment? This is a stark uncertainty of self for Dr Clarke.

Summary

Dr Clarke has encountered considerable difficulty in reaching a decision in a perplexing case. Not only has he found uncertainty over which set of diagnostic criteria he ought to use, but his introspection, coupled with his conversations with colleagues, has uncovered ethical and legal uncertainties along with perturbing uncertainties of interpretation and personal integrity. The doctor has set aside precious time from a busy week to reflect explicitly about these complexities. This has made him acutely aware that he might evoke a similar process of deliberation for every patient he sees, and that if he did this he would be unable to offer practical help to anybody. Dr Clarke would like to feel absolutely confident about the decision in Shirley's case, but he now recognises that he cannot achieve this level of certainty. He feels that there is much more to this issue than first appeared, and he wishes that he had some clear guide to help him recognise his most appropriate role.

The beginnings of a broader argument

Beyond the particular concerns of Dr Clarke the stage has been set for a broader argument. It has been asserted that any medical intervention must meet uncertainty of some kind at some stage. However, some may feel that the example of anorexia nervosa is simply too convenient for this claim to be convincing. It might be objected that anorexia is an exceptional, atypical, medical problem and that there are far more and far deeper uncertainties in this case than with most clinical work. Such an example loads the dice. To have real merit the idea that uncertainty pervades medicine should be tested against hard cases—physical ailments, such as oesophageal carcinoma, ruptured spleen and gonorrhoea, which are clearly defined, their treatments carefully researched and objectively presented.

This potential complaint is acknowledged. In the following chapter the example of hypertension is considered. This common medical problem is found to raise the same categories of uncertainty as anorexia nervosa. In addition, throughout this book there are examples of standard medical cases and activities, all of which exhibit various aspects of uncertainty. It will become clear that in order to find the most satisfactory solutions to medical problems it is necessary to recognise the full range of types of persisting uncertainty.

Chapter Two

What Is Normal?

Medical work, whatever its context, must inevitably meet uncertainty of some kind at some point. Whether the encounter occurs early—during diagnosis—or later—during therapy—there will be an aspect of the task which cannot be tackled solely by precise clinical science.

Uncertainty runs deep in medicine. This chapter introduces the most fundamental uncertainty. It is an abiding source of imprecision, an uncertainty at the heart of medical work. It is uncertainty over what is and what is not to count as *normal*. Normality cannot simply be observed. Somebody has to decide whether something counts as normal or not. This does not mean that medicine cannot employ exacting scientific measurement to good effect, but it does imply that a range of human forces shape medicine's view of normality—and so shape medicine. Politics, culture, class, race, gender, and personal preference each have a part to play in structuring medical activity. These forces have been analysed extensively in medical sociology, and so are not singled out for special attention in this chapter. Instead the examples of statistics and law are used to show that medicine should never be thought of as a purely objective activity.

Bringing 'Normals' into Question

Traditionally medical students and doctors have been encouraged to take certain features of medical practice for granted, as being simply true and needing neither further investigation nor confirmation. For example, few doubts are raised in medical schools that drug therapy should be central to good medicine, or that quantitative methods are the way to assess people's health status. Perhaps the least examined assumption in current medical education is the belief that practitioners should aim to prevent or cure abnormality: it is apparently a quite basic belief in medicine that the continuation or restoration of normality is a primary goal. As students progress through their training, and as doctors develop in their careers, it is expected that they will accumulate a growing body of knowledge about normal and abnormal conditions, and in the process become ever more adept at identifying deviations from 'the norm'. Normality seems to be the first touchstone of medicine. However, when the *idea* of 'normal' and 'abnormal' is thought about carefully, whether in the abstract or with reference to practical examples, it is soon clear that decisions about what is and is not normal have some degree of arbitrariness about them.

It can be a salutary yet ultimately enlightening process for doctors to question the standard judgements of normality which they encounter daily in their work.

Genuinely worrying about the question 'what is normal' will inevitably generate confusion—a feeling which is invariably coupled with frustration, unease at what seems to be an unnecessary complication of an essentially practical enterprise—disease management and the care of patients. But reflection about the nature of normality can also produce great benefit. Doggedly puzzling over the limits of normality can eventually clear the conceptual ground, can help clarify the *raison d'etre* of medicine, leaving room for a fresh interpretation of the discipline's basic purpose. The insight spawned by pressing the question *'What is normal in medicine?'* to a logical conclusion can inspire new thinking about the richest, most creative forms of practical intervention.

Differing Normals

Normality has been claimed for an incredible variety of states and activities. 'This is normal' must have been said at one time or another of almost every imaginable event and practice—from wrapping corpses in preservatives and placing them in vast tombs surrounded by fantastic wealth, to sitting in front of a box of electronics watching Leslie Crowther and Cilla Black play games on a Saturday night.

Any casual survey of everyday conversation and writing quickly turns up phrases in which 'normal' is used in different ways. For example, it is common to hear or read discussions of 'normal attitudes', 'statistical norms', 'normal appearance', or 'normal practice', and to recognise that different meanings are intended. For instance a British Muslim might praise abstinence from alcohol as a 'normal attitude' whereas the 'statistical norm' of alcohol consumption in all British adults is that the majority drink alcohol sometimes. In this example the uses of normal are primarily distinguished by the fact that the former is infused with value, and the latter is simply descriptive. The Muslim uses 'normal' to transmit approval of a certain practice, whereas the statistician merely reports an observed correlation.

How do you find a normal person?

Imagine your boss asking you to go out and talk to a 'normal' person. It is likely that unless she happens to be editor of a tabloid newspaper you will think she has become deranged overnight, since without definition the task is impossible.

Any practical research into normality must always assume certain standards as given, and must be carried out in specified contexts. The question *'What is normal?'* asked in the abstract is quite meaningless. If you are asked out of the blue by a stranger, *'What is normal?'*, you might either ignore the question (which would seem to be the most sensible option, particularly if you are asked this at the start of an *Intercity* train ride) or ask in turn, 'What do you mean? Which subject do you want my opinion on?' In order to answer the question at all both the type of normality to be considered and the area under discussion must be described. The original question must be given body, perhaps like this, 'What I mean is, when in Spain, what is normal as regards eating times and habits?' Only at this point can meaningful conversation begin.

Considered at the most superficial level most people are by definition 'normal' in that they are unremarkable. Thought of in this weak sense a 'normal person' is the girl sitting opposite you on the train to work, the joking middle-aged man who collects your ticket, the boy on his skate-board performing tricks on the slope outside the station, and the severe grey-haired man who nods at you, you suspect a little resentfully, as you overtake him on the stairs to your floor at work. However, if the question '*Is this person normal or not?*' is pressed further, if the categories under examination are specified more precisely certain difficulties emerge. At any level deeper than '*man-in-the-street normality*', whether each person qualifies as normal or not becomes more difficult to say. Is the assessment of normality to concern age, income, physiological state, sexuality, hobbies, political viewpoint, or some other variable?

The girl on the train is pregnant, which in one sense is not the 'normal' condition of the female adult population. But the pregnancy is 'normal' in another sense, in that it has developed typically so far. The ticket collector suffers pain as the result of an old football injury, he suffers hayfever every summer, cannot go a day without a drink, but never misses a day at his post. Should he be described as generally normal or abnormal? The boy has a nagging tooth-ache, he masturbates daily, and he suffers the occasional migraine headache. Is it correct to say that he is entirely normal, or would it be better to conclude that he is partly abnormal? The severe grey-haired man is stressed: he has high blood pressure, he feels intensely awkward in his body, he is unable to make small-talk, and he avoids people if at all possible. Is he abnormal on all counts, or is still further detail required for an authoritative opinion? It is very hard to say, and it does not become an easier task with the addition of greater detail. The following example shows that even high precision will not necessarily resolve the issue.

Hypertension: An Example from the Core of Medicine

The fact that the notion of 'normality' is so ambiguous is not merely a philosophical worry. It is not an issue of only peripheral concern, something to mull over during an idle moment. On the contrary, deciding what normality is can pose central practical difficulties for medicine.

The example of hypertension displays both the reality of the conundrum, and the importance that a doctor's interpretation of the question, '*What is normal?*' can have for patients. Dependent upon a doctor's decision about whether a blood-pressure reading falls inside or outside a range or normality a patient can find himself left alone, or placed on a potentially harmful therapeutic regime. The doctor finds herself walking a tightrope. Not only must she decide whether to treat or not, and how to treat, she must also make a careful prior decision about the extent of the range of normality. Should she choose a narrow range of 'normal', so making sure of finding many abnormals (just in case!), or should she choose a large range of 'normal', so ensuring that the abnormals she finds truly warrant her valuable time and attention?

Unlike anorexia nervosa, which is a relatively rare condition [16], hypertension is a common problem in medicine. Hodgkin [17] reports a national incidence of 22.4 patients per thousand per year. On top of this he speculates that recent screening programmes may have doubled or trebled this figure.

Background

Hypertension is generally associated with increased liability to coronary artery disease, cerebrovascular accident, heart failure and peripheral vascular disease. There is little doubt about the causal significance of established diastolic hypertension, although the evidence against systolic or mild diastolic elevation is less emphatic, despite a number of large-scale studies of intervention*. In clinical practice this uncertainty becomes manifest in disagreements between doctors over the correct definition of mild and moderate hypertension. The practical implication of this is that different clinicians will choose different levels of blood pressure as points at which to intervene with patients. Thus, far from being an 'armchair problem', a decision about what counts as 'normal' can have a crucial effect on the life of another person. The decision can be particularly significant if long-term drug treatment is contemplated.

The uncertainty is deepened by the knowledge that blood pressure can be affected by the circumstances, the equipment, and the personnel involved in its measurement. It is recognised that raised blood pressure can occur in the presence of a doctor purely as a result of anxiety, and not at any other time. This effect is known as 'white-coat' or 'office' hypertension. In recent studies, between 10% and 30% of hospital patients with hypertension fell into this category. Evidence is accumulating that continuous blood pressure measurement over a 24-hour period provides closer correlation with end-organ damage than single readings, thus calling into question the reliability of casual monitoring [18–28].**

Exercise One

This is the first of eight exercises. Each has been designed for use either by the reader in private, or by groups in an organised class. The basic point of each exercise is to allow the player to experience uncertainty, to experience how uncertainty might feel to other people, and to begin to think of ways to deal with it.

Pressures

Characters

Dr Jenkins
Christopher

Select one of these characters, either the doctor or the patient. Read the scenario as it unfolds, and try to imagine how you would feel if you were that character. Also reflect upon the considerable uncertainty with which either character must deal.

Each of the uncertainties discussed in Chapter One are present.

continued on next page

---

*Diastolic refers to the pressure of blood in the arteries during the relaxed phase. Systolic refers to the highest point of the pressure.
**The term end-organ damage refers to structures with a vascular bed connected to the arterial system. The arterioles become damaged as a result of high blood pressure. In this way the eyes and kidneys, for instance, can function less well or fail completely.

continued

A sleek 38-year-old marketing executive called Christopher has just had some bad news. He has attended a clinic away from his usual health centre in order to have a pre-employment medical for a job which means a considerable promotion and jump in salary. Christopher has been told that his blood pressure is 180/110, and that this is clearly not normal. It was explained that his readings are cause for concern, but that immediate action is not essential. Even if it is not right to describe him as ill at the moment, there is a strong and definite risk of future illness.

As he drives home in his BMW (a car leased to him by his present employer), he wonders how Julia will react, and what the children might think. Julia will be sick, she'll worry that he'll lose the new job. Perhaps he won't tell her. Perhaps the doctor was wrong. Perhaps the equipment was faulty. Doesn't blood pressure vary? Perhaps it will be lower if he takes further tests. Three nights jogging a week, not overweight, no smoking, drinking regularly but never drunk—a man in his prime: surely there has been a mistake. He decides not to tell Julia, but to keep quiet for the time being. If he does tell her he knows there is a chance that the situation might become more stressful for him.

Christopher visits his general practitioner, Dr Jenkins, in order to sort the thing out. He hands the doctor the results of his check-up, and immediately regales him with a numbingly detailed account of his fitness, his abstinence from tobacco, his 81 minutes in the Little Wittering Ten, his mantra, and his 'Hill Climber' exerciser. Christopher ends with the plea, 'Please test me again, Doctor, I'm a normal healthy man'. Relieved to be free of the verbal pressure to declare the businessman normal, before any clinical intervention on his part, Dr Jenkins does the test. On this occasion the reading is 170/95, it has come down significantly but in Jenkins's opinion is not normal. Christopher's blood pressure remains cause for concern.

If Christopher were to have his blood pressure measured in America, it is probable that this reading would trigger an intervention. In the USA doctors tend to intervene at lower pressures [29].

Christopher responds with some satisfaction, 'Isn't this much better though? I feel great. I can't see that I have anything to worry about?' Measuring his words, his doctor replies that most doctors accept a range of normality in men in his age-group. In the UK, this is around 140/90 while in the USA around 130/80. Christopher jumps at this: 'How can you accept that? If doctors disagree so much, how can you expect me to take your word for it that I'm not normal?' Dr Jenkins acknowledges calmly that there is a level of controversy in medical circles over the subject of hypertension. However, some pressures, such as 180/110—Christopher's original reading—are clearly out of the ordinary. All doctors would agree that such a reading is cause for some concern. He goes on to explain that a person's blood pressure will vary over the course of the day, and may be affected by the circumstances in which it is taken. For instance, anxiety can significantly increase blood pressure for a short period. It may be that Christopher finds having his blood pressure taken a stressful experience, and that he may have found his pre-employment medical particularly nerve-wracking. Because of this uncertainty Dr Jenkins suggests that it would be sensible to take Christopher's blood pressure on three further occasions over the next few weeks, in order to obtain the truest picture.

continued on next page

continued

Two months later, Christopher has not given a reading lower than 160/90. Dr Jenkins suggests to him that it is time to face the facts, and to consider the various treatment options. But Christopher, who has not been able to take up his new job because of the doubt over his health, asserts that he feels fine. He's very fit, he says. Arrogantly, he challenges the flabby 32-year-old Jenkins to a race over five miles. Of course he's 'effing' normal. The situation has become very tense between the doctor and patient.

Christopher demands a second opinion, but Dr Jenkins is reluctant to refer him. So, angry and upset, Christopher privately arranges a test and interview with a consultant. The test is carried out and produces a reading of 170/95, but Christopher is obviously tense. The consultant tells Christopher not to worry because he is 'probably alright', and says he will write to Dr Jenkins with the result.

NETHERLEY GENERAL HOSPITAL
NETHERFIELD ROAD
NETHERLEY
MELCHESTER

3rd January 1990

Dr R Jenkins
Larkhill Health Centre,
Hawthorn Road,
Larkhill,
Melchester.

Dear Dr Jenkins

I have seen Mr Christopher Smythe-Hennessey today and found his blood pressure to be 170/95. I have ascertained that there is no evidence of end-organ damage. I have discussed his eating, drinking, exercise and work patterns with him. In my opinion, atenolol might in the circumstances be appropriate. However, I could also understand a policy of non-intervention. I must leave the final judgement in your hands.

Yours sincerely,

Michael Bates,
Consultant Physician

At this point Christopher has had several readings that are probably abnormal, and none in the range accepted as being clearly normal. Although each reading could be said to be within the 'grey' borderline area, the consistency of result persuades Dr Jenkins that a positive intervention is required. The general practitioner is aware that as a prerequisite, as a necessary first step towards further intervention, it remains necessary to convince Christopher that he is not 'perfectly normal'. If this can be achieved then fresh options become available to Dr Jenkins and Christopher.

continued on next page

continued

Options

Simply, the options are:

(1) to carry out further tests (such as 24-hour monitoring) to establish that a problem exists and what its cause might be;
(2) to suggest that the patient is merely observed . . . 'we'll just keep an eye on you';
(3) to suggest immediate drug intervention to reduce the blood pressure;
(4) to suggest immediate non-drug intervention, for instance, behaviour change, bio-feedback or yoga might be helpful [30].

Role play/thought play

Now either play out, or imagine how you would play out, the consultation in which Dr Jenkins changes his role from one of fairly gentle, supportive adviser to one of a doctor striving for patient compliance. Christopher, at least at first, continues to resist.

It might be helpful to know that further tests might include a cardiograph taken by the consultant; a search for rare causes of the raised blood pressure through 24-hour urine collection, intravenous pyelogram (for renal artery stenosis), or serum electrolytes (to test for a benign tumour of the adrenals). If drug therapy is recommended, this may cause unwanted effects such as tiredness or impotence. Dr Jenkins will have to decide whether or not Christopher should be told of these possible difficulties. Will the possibility of impotence make his compliance with drug therapy even less likely?

Whether you are Christopher or Dr Jenkins, it is important to reach a view about whether or not Christopher is actually ill. And, if Christopher is ill, does this reduce his status in any way? For instance, is his competence to make decisions reduced? In what sense might his competence be reduced? Is there any possibility of heightening his competence? If his status and competence is diminished in some way does Dr Jenkins have a duty to do whatever he thinks is in Christopher's best interest? Does Dr Jenkins have the right to put other pressures on Christopher—to persuade, to coerce, or even to frighten him about the possible consequences of doing nothing?

Perhaps the central questions are these: What is the priority for Dr Jenkins? What is the priority for Christopher? Are these the same? What ought their priorities to be?

Pervasive uncertainty

If it were possible to state unequivocally that between measurement X and measurement Y blood pressure is always normal and presents no problems, and that beyond that range intervention is always correct and desirable, there would be no uncertainty. However, a world in which a statement such as this would be possible would be a very different place from the one we inhabit. Since our world is imperfect it is inevitable that uncertainty will be present. One way to manage this uncertainty is to categorise it into standard formats. The key question remains, *'Should I intervene, and, if so, how?'*

To draw a parallel with the anorexia nervosa study, the *first uncertainty* (the uncertainty of diagnosis) might be said to be this. Firstly, can blood pressure be used—on its own or even at all—to diagnose accurately a problematic physiological condition (What is normal blood pressure? What ranges will different individuals tolerate?). Secondly, does the method of measurement (whatever type it is) give an accurate picture of a person's continuous blood pressure?

In any case of suspected hypertension there will be uncertainty about which method of treatment to apply. For example, should drugs be used immediately or should changes to 'life-style' be attempted first? Or should nothing be done? Different doctors will prefer different solutions. This uncertainty can be reduced by intelligent attention to personal and family history, and by analysis of the probable outcomes of the different types of intervention, but it cannot be reduced entirely to certainty.

One *ethical uncertainty* (and there are many) hinges on the issues of what advice is given, how it is delivered, and whether or not drug treatment is prescribed. For example, if the hypertensive is a 48-year-old man with a mean diastolic pressure of 100 mmHg who drinks 8 to 10 units of alcohol per day, smokes 10 cigarettes daily, and enjoys this way of life—do you offer him the option of reducing his smoking and drinking? (is the problem one requiring only simple, harmless education?), do you try to frighten him? do you insist that the essential target must be to reduce his blood pressure? Or do you consider the curtailment of his enjoyment not to be a price worth paying, even taking into account the increased risk of the man using up scarce health service resources if his condition does not improve? Since anxiety and stress have been shown to increase levels of blood pressure, should information be kept to a minimum, and is a more paternalist drug-based intervention preferred instead? In other words, a balancing of costs may have to be considered. Are the side-effects of the drugs less harmful than the effect of raising a person's anxiety? Or is there a greater cost to be paid in terms of loss of patient autonomy? Can these costs be balanced at all, or are they incommensurable? Is it impossible to compare them meaningfully?

In the case of hypertension there is no immediate *legal uncertainty* so long as the patient consents to his blood pressure being monitored, and so long as this is done properly, but *uncertainty of interpretation* and *self* are probable.

One *uncertainty of interpretation* may stem from a puzzle about whether it is correct to interpret most hypertension as a problem at all. It is probably correct to say:

> 'On present evidence in Britain at least 4% of men and 5.5% of women aged 35 to 64 would probably prolong their lives and reduce their risks of crippling by stroke, by receiving continuing antihypertensive treatment [31].'

But what is *not clear* is why this should be ultimately so important. What is a 'healthy life'? The answer is far from obvious.

The doctor's image of a healthy life might not be the image held by the patient of the life she wants. Long-term medication is not everybody's idea of fun. And if the unprovable is assumed, if it is taken to be true that Tudor Hart's interpretation of a 'healthy life' is crucially important—in other words that longevity and freedom from the problems associated with high blood pressure are *imperatives*—then is the doctor not morally obliged to take other steps to ensure these imperatives such as insisting that his patients exercise for half an hour three times a week?

An *uncertainty of self* in the case of hypertension might occur if the doctor doubts whether his intervention is justified. Given the *first uncertainty* over the definition of abnormal blood pressure, and about how best to obtain an accurate picture, should a doctor test blood pressure at all if this will generate only anxiety and further uncertainty? For instance, if the pressure is likely to turn out to be only a few points above the accepted highest point is it worth causing the worry to the patient? Can the doctor achieve anything worthwhile by taking blood pressure? Does he have a legitimate and worthwhile role? Will he simply be doing more harm than good?

Shifting normals

As can be seen from the puzzle which surrounds hypertensive illness, because the term 'normal' can be used in different ways it is quite possible for the same object or event to be described simultaneously as both 'normal' and 'abnormal' if different standards are chosen. Christopher regards his physical state as normal because he can detect no difference between the way he feels now and the way he has felt when he was defined as healthy in the past. But the doctors are applying a different norm—normality assessed for populations. On this standard rather than his individual standard, Christopher falls outside the range of normality.

The issue of what is normal is at the hub of the quandary over certainty in both the example of anorexia nervosa and hypertension. By nature and profession, doctors are doers. They must act, and cannot afford to worry for too long about the nature of normality when faced with sickness. But clinicians do have quieter moments, and it is during this time that deliberation about the source of standards and norms can pay rich dividends. It is important to explore the issue of normality a little further before moving on to demonstrate that normality must be at least partially *created*.

Normality is not a static thing. Normality changes as a river changes dependent upon the terrain over which it flows. What counts as normal changes over life-times and cultures, sometimes with bewildering frequency. In young children the defined range of normality for many aspects moves rapidly. For example, after birth a baby's haemoglobin level falls quickly over a period of weeks. During the childhood years expected weight, height and head circumference alter at different rates, the various aspects changing independently, not in parallels. Consequently, any assessment of normality in childhood cannot refer to a single standard. Instead, any standard selected must specify both the age limits within which to calculate and the specific aspects of the child or children to be assessed.

In middle-aged and elderly people the accepted ranges of statistical normality show that the idea of normality can simply make no sense if it is thought of as fixed. For example, vision and hearing tend to deteriorate, which is 'normal' in older age groups, but not 'normal' in younger people. Normality shifts with age. In older people what counts as 'normal' for the age group is sometimes thought to require medical treatment.

In multiracial communities ethnic factors can alter defined ranges of normality. For example, an eosinophil* count of 9% may well be considered 'normal' amongst Pakistani children coming to live in Britain. Similarly the range of 'normal' for height, weight and head circumference amongst Nigerian children can be markedly different from their peers of European origin. Ranges of normality are not permanently fixed; normality is not constantly hooked to the same place in reality—the notion of normality is not solid but fluid.

Review

To sum up so far, it has become apparent that the further the question '*What is normal?*' is probed, the more confusing it becomes. It would be possible to undertake a detailed, and inevitably lengthy, philosophical clarification of the range of meanings and uses of the word 'normal'. Understanding of 'normality' as a notion or set of theories might improve as a result, but this book is intended to be primarily of practical help—to equip doctors with an understanding of the reality of uncertainty, and to suggest ways of coping with it. With this in mind, the following section introduces two of the major forces which shape the medical view of normality.

These forces are statistics and law, and they shape medical reality in different ways. Statistics help doctors pinpoint the ranges of states and conditions which can be measured and defined numerically (although it is well worth remembering that such states and conditions are by no means all there is to the human experience). Law, on the other hand, tends to empower doctors in another fashion. Legal judgements help shape what counts as normal acceptable medical practice. In addition to the rulings of the courts, Acts of Parliament have extended the role of doctors in certain areas, granting the power to medics to take decisions in areas of life that can hardly be described as clinical.

However, neither of these forces works entirely objectively, entirely apart from opinion. In both cases human judgement works to fashion those things which are taken to be normal. Because of this—because even statistics and law, which are commonly believed to be rigid arbiters, can offer no absolute authority—medicine must accept uncertainty. The discipline must countenance the truth that its very being depends in part upon personal judgement.

In Chapter Three, where the notions of disease and health are dissected, the presence of this inescapable element of subjective judgement is found to have far-reaching implications for medical practice—especially for those doctors who regard their work as essentially work for health. However, the subjective element within statistics and law must first be revealed.

Forces Shaping Normality in Medicine

Statistics and 'normality'

In medicine 'statistical norms' are thought to be essential for formal research.

---

*Eosinophil is any cell in the body with granules in its substance that stain easily with the dye eosin. About 2% of white blood cells are eosinophils. Eosinophil cells are also present in the pituitary gland.

Eosinophilia means an 'abnormal' increase in the number of eosinophils in the blood. It occurs in Hodgkin's disease, asthma, hay fever, some skin diseases, and parasitic infestations [32].

Results of clinical research are said to be interesting when tests show significant deviations from expected or established norms. For instance, if the reactions of human subjects taking a particular drug are tested against those of control groups taking other drugs or placebos, and their responses are found to be significantly better than the mean, then this will probably be regarded as a contribution to medical knowledge, and fresh help in the fight against a particular disease.

Statistically inspired definitions of normality are frequently used by doctors in daily practice with individual patients. Certain 'norms' are implied in height and weight charts, haematology reports and blood-pressure readings. Naturally doctors make use of these standards in diagnosis and treatment, but the fact that they are often found to be useful does not mean that they are written on tablets of stone—the standards are questionable and open to challenge. Every measurable feature of human beings varies from individual to individual. And even when single individuals are the sole subjects of measurement, readings of particular aspects of them can show a wide range of 'scatter' or 'dispersion', as is often the case with blood pressure.

The doctor must make a decision about where the cut-off point between normality and abnormality is to lie. If she wishes to define the statistical limits to normality for any particular feature she wishes to measure the doctor has to select:

(1) The core value (which statisticians call the 'central tendency') on which the range of normality for that aspect is to be centred.
(2) The range of values (on either side of the chosen core value) which she will regard as 'normal', and the place where the limit is reached.

But how is she to do this with certainty?

One basic option in statistics

In order to decide upon the 'central tendency' the doctor might employ either the Mean, Mode or Median measurement. The *arithmetic mean* is the sum of the measurements divided by the number of measurements; the *mode* is the measurement occurring most frequently; and the *median* is the measurement which lies in the middle when all the measurements are ranked in order of value—the central value, with an equal number of observations larger and smaller than itself.

But these measurements can produce different results. To take an example from a clinical textbook [33]:

'. . . suppose that 70 female patients, consulting with a lump in the breast, show varying delays between noticing and reporting the lump:

Delays in weeks, up to:	1	2	3	4	5	6	7	8	9	10	11	12	13	14	15	16	17	18
No. of patients:		5	6	10	12	8	6	2	5	2	4	3	0	2	0	1	1	2	1

What is to be regarded as the 'normal' delay period for such consultations? If the doctor plots the delays on a graph, he will obtain a curve which is skewed to the left. Here the Mean (6.0), the Mode (4) and the Median (5) no longer coincide; and in distribution curves with a 'positive skew':

Mean > Median > Mode'

Leading statisticians readily acknowledge that there is an arbitrary element in labelling measurements 'normal' and 'abnormal'. The accepted method of establishing numerical norms is to take a sample of 'healthy' people and to define 2.5% at either end of the spectrum as 'abnormal'. In other words, to define 5% of the sample as simultaneously 'normal' and 'abnormal'. Statisticians have commented that:

> 'The misleading phrase "normal limits" for physiologic measurements has generally been interpreted as a pair of numbers such that 95% of measurements made on healthy persons fall between these numbers, and 2½% fall on each side. The absurdity of the use of the words "normal" and "abnormal" with reference to these percentage points is obvious.' [34]

The difficulty for the doctor who aspires to certainty is that even in the simplest case where he hopes to arrive at an assessment of normality by the use of statistics there is not *one* 'normal' but there are several. He must make a choice and he cannot turn ultimately to statistics for certainty, for this will be a circular ploy, and he will succeed only in revolving to another point where he must choose. Eventually he will have to make a judgement, the basis of which will involve a number of factors—some measurable and some not. However much detail is explored in statistics the picture is, once again, one of uncertainty in an area of inquiry where one might reasonably have expected certainty.

Statistics is only one of many forces which shape normality in medicine. Although statistical techniques are not imposed on medicine, and although they seem to be merely innocuous mathematical devices to aid clinical understanding, they none the less reflect a degree of personal judgement. At the other end of the spectrum, where medicine falls within the scrutiny of law, the presence of human opinion becomes more strikingly apparent.

Law shaping medicine: the 'reasonable doctor' is the normal doctor

Basic background

There are two primary sources of law in England. Law can be created by Statute enacted by Parliament, and by judgements made in court cases. It is in these court cases that judges create the 'common law' of England. Their verdicts can set precedents which may be the only authority which exists in certain categories of law. Much medical law is made in this way. It is possible for Parliament to legislate to change the law decided in a court case, and to this extent court cases are subordinate to the rule of Parliament. In addition, courts must follow decisions made by courts superior in the hierarchy of law—so the Court of Appeal sets the standard for the High Court, and is in turn governed by judgements made in the House of Lords. The House of Lords can in certain circumstances decide not to follow a decision made previously.

The law is now regularly called upon to arbitrate in disputes over what is, or is not, good medical care. Current law can change as judges make new rulings in fresh cases. Such rulings often seem to be a balance between legal and medical opinion as to what counts as acceptable practice.

There are several good textbooks available on the law as it relates to medicine [35, 36, 37], and such comprehensive material is not reproduced here.

Shaping the 'reasonable doctor'

By finding the practice of some doctors to be negligent the law acts as one limit on medical activity. It is up to the plaintiff (the aggrieved person bringing the action) to prove, on the balance of probabilities, that a doctor has been negligent. In order to do this the plaintiff must establish three points:

(1) that the doctor owed him a duty of care (that the doctor had an obligation to exercise caution);
(2) that the duty was breached; and
(3) that he suffered harm caused by that breach.

Once a precedent has been set in case law then a doctor can expect that if he acts in a similar way to a defendant previously found to be negligent, then it is possible that he will be sued, and might lose the case.

This is one example of a successful claim in negligence, a claim which satisfied the above three conditions.

'Cassidy v Ministry of Health
[1951] 2KB 343, [1951] 1 All ER 574, CA
The plaintiff entered hospital for an operation on his left hand. At the end of post-operative treatment his hand was made worse. He sued the Minister responsible for the hospital. The Court of Appeal allowed an appeal by the plaintiff and held the hospital authority liable.

Denning LJ: *Turning now to the facts in this case, this is the position: the hospital authorities accepted the patient for treatment, and it was their duty to treat him with reasonable care. They selected, employed and paid all the surgeons and nurses who looked after him. He had no say in their selection at all. If those surgeons and nurses did not treat him with proper care and skill, then the hospital authorities must answer for it, for it means that they themselves did not perform their duty to him.'* [38].

This case was won against a hospital authority, but it is quite clear that doctors must take care not to overstep the limits on their practice set down in law. However, the law is not an impartial referee. In fact, the law allows doctors considerable power to shape their roles within the various civil and criminal legal limits which exist. Doctors themselves, in very many cases, are permitted to be the arbiters of what is reasonable—of what is normal medical practice. As Margaret Brazier has written:

'The judges in England defer in the most part to the views of the doctors . . . English judges will rarely challenge the accepted views of the medical profession. Establishing what that view is may cause the court some difficulty though. Each side is free to call its own experts and a clash of eminent medical opinion is not unusual.' [39]

Two cases are particularly relevant to demonstrate the power that medical judgement has over standards of normal practice, at least in Great Britain.

Bolam v Friern Hospital Management Committee
[1957] 2 All ER 118, [1957] 1 WLR 582

Facts: The plaintiff contended that the defendants were vicariously liable for the carelessness of a doctor who administered electro-convulsive therapy to the plaintiff without administering a relaxant drug or without restraining the convulsive movements of the plaintiff by manual control (save for his lower jaw). The plaintiff suffered a fractured jaw as a consequence. He brought an action against the defendants in negligence.

McNair J directed the jury:

I must explain what in law we mean by 'negligence'. In the ordinary case which does not involve any special skill, negligence in law means this: Some failure to do some act which a reasonable man in the circumstances would do, or doing some act which a reasonable man in the circumstances would not do; and if that failure or doing of that act results in injury, then there is a cause of action.

. . . But the emphasis which is laid by counsel for the defendants is on this aspect of negligence: He submitted to you that the real question on which you have to make up your mind on each of the three major points to be considered is whether the defendants, in acting in the way in which they did, were acting in accordance with a practice of competent respected professional opinion. Counsel for the defendants submitted that if you are satisfied that they were acting in accordance with a practice of a competent body of professional opinion, then it would be wrong for you to hold that negligence was established

. . . I myself would prefer to put it this way: A doctor is not guilty of negligence if he has acted in accordance with a practice accepted as proper by a responsible body of medical men skilled in that particular art. I do not think there is much difference in sense. It is just a different way of expressing the same thought. Putting it the other way round, a doctor is not negligent, if he is acting in accordance with such a practice, merely because there is a body of opinion that takes a contrary view. At the same time, that does not mean that a medical man can obstinately and pig-headedly carry on with some old technique if it has been proved to be contrary to what is really substantially the whole of informed medical opinion. Otherwise you might get men today saying: "I don't believe in anaesthetics. I don't believe in antiseptics. I am going to continue to do my surgery in the way it was done in the eighteenth century". That clearly would be wrong.

The jury returned a verdict for the defendants.' [40]

This case established what is known as the 'Bolam Test', or 'the reasonable doctor test'. As the law stands, if a doctor can produce evidence that a 'responsible body of medical men skilled in that particular art' would have acted as he acted, then there can be no ground for an action in negligence. Normal practice, it is held, cannot by definition be negligent. As Lord Scarman commented in the Sidaway Case:

'*The Bolam principle may be formulated as a rule that a doctor is not negligent if he acts in accordance with a practice accepted at the time as proper by a responsible body of medical opinion even though other doctors adopt a different practice. In short, the law imposes the duty of care; but the standard of care is a matter of medical judgement.*' [41]

With the help of the law, doctors set the standard of normal practice. The Sidaway case is controversial not only because it confirms the 'Bolam Test', but also because it allows doctors rather than patients to be the ultimate judges of what information should be conveyed. It is quoted at length because it is discussed later in the book, in the light of philosophical rather than legal discussion.

'*Sidaway v Board of Governors of the Bethlem Royal Hospital*
[1985] AC 871, [1985] 1 All ER 643

Facts: The plaintiff, who had suffered recurrent pain in her neck, right shoulder and arms, underwent an operation in 1974 which was performed by a senior neurosurgeon at the first defendant's hospital. The operation, even if performed with proper care and skill, carried an inherent material risk, which was put at between one and two per cent, of damage to the spinal column and the nerve roots. The risk of damage to the spinal column was substantially less than to a nerve root but the consequences were much more serious. In consequence of the operation the plaintiff was severely disabled. Her monetary loss was assessed at £67,500.

The plaintiff claimed damages for negligence against the hospital and the executors of the deceased surgeon, the second defendants. She relied solely on the alleged failure of the surgeon to disclose or explain to her the risks inherent in, or special to, the operation which he had advised. Skinner J found that the surgeon did not tell the plaintiff that it was an operation of choice rather than necessity; that whilst he had told her of the possibility of disturbing a nerve root and the consequences, he did not refer to the danger of damage to the spinal cord; that in refraining from informing her of those two factors he was following a practice which in 1974 would have been accepted as proper by a responsible body of skilled and experienced neurosurgeons; and applying the test formulated in *Bolam v Friern Management Committee* [1957] 1 WLR 582 that the standard of care was that of the ordinary skilled man exercising and professing to have that special skill and that a doctor was not negligent if he acted in accordance with the practice accepted at the time as proper by a responsible body of medical opinion, notwithstanding that other doctors adopted different practices, the judge dismissed the plaintiff's claim. The Court of Appeal affirmed Skinner J's decision.' [42]

Despite a dissenting verdict which aimed to establish that, regardless of the views of a 'responsible body of medical opinion', the patient has a right to know of the material risks of an operation, it remains the case that if a body of opinion can be found to support the action of the doctor accused of negligence then, on the application of the 'Bolam Test', the plaintiff will fail.

Thus the judges and the doctors both contribute to the establishment of what is to count as normal practice, and what the limits on normal practice ought to be. Once again it can be seen that the setting of norms depends upon human judgement. Always there are factors in play which are external to judgement—What are the facts of the case? What is the extent of the injury? But unless a human decision is made about where to draw the line *there can be no standards at all*.

This insight is crucial to this inquiry. It has major ramifications for both the goals and the conduct of medical practice. In order to show how important human perception of normal and abnormal is, it is necessary to take three further careful steps. These are firstly to accept that not even the description of human physical and mental conditions as diseases is an entirely objective judgement. Even to describe a cancer as a disease carries with it an element of human bias. And then to accept that if this is so diseases cannot be regarded as special, unique and separate problems of human life, but as obstacles of the same general sort as any other obstacle to states of existence which human beings desire. Given these two steps it is then possible legitimately to discard the view that medicine should be concerned only with problems directly associated with disease. This third step has far-reaching implications for the future organisation and delivery of health care.

It is necessary to advance the argument in this studied manner because although the steps may appear to be mundane and obvious to some if taken separately, when they are considered at once they can be genuinely surprising. The conclusions which follow from the accumulated steps are controversial. It is crucial to show that they are not sweeping generalisations, but can be shown to have developed logically, as the result of dispassionate analysis.

Exercise Two

Scarred for Life?

The characters

Alan Smith (aged 22, professional ice-hockey player)
Dr Pearce (GP and Mersey Falcons' doctor)
Mr Brooks (solicitor)
Mr Gavins (plastic surgeon)
Professor Peterson (GP expert witness)

The situation

Alan Smith is proposing to sue Dr Pearce for negligence. He believes that he has a good case, and that he ought to receive some compensation for his injury, for his loss of earnings and for the damage done to his career. Mr Brooks is Alan Smith's solicitor.

When he was thirteen Alan Smith was vaccinated against tuberculosis (BCG vaccination) prior to travelling abroad on a school trip. The vaccination caused his arm to swell and it left a small but unsightly swelling and scar on his left arm. The scar was not painful, but Alan was aware of its unpleasant appearance when sun-bathing or when swimming. His doctor advised Alan and his mother that no treatment was necessary. On his eighteenth birthday Alan signed as an apprentice for Mersey Falcons. During the medical examination Dr Pearce noticed the swelling and scar, and asked Alan to attend the following day so that he could 'deal with it'. He told Alan that it would be a minor matter to cut out the swelling and scar. Alan thought little of this. He was satisfied that the doctor knew best, and he was keen to do anything that the people at Mersey Falcons wished—it was his first professional ice-hockey appointment.

The next day Alan arrived at the doctor's surgery. Dr Pearce explained again that he was simply going to cut away the swelling and the scar, and would then stitch up the small wound which would heal, eventually to leave only a negligible scar.

continued on next page

continued

Alan did not sign a consent form to the operation which was carried out under local anaesthetic. Afterwards Alan noticed that the wound was much longer (3 inches) than he had imagined from Dr Pearce's account, and that there were twelve stitches. He showed his shoulder to his mother, an ex-nurse. She was also surprised by the extent of the surgery, and she noticed that the middle of the wound did not meet. This seemed to be due to the natural tension created by Alan's well-muscled shoulder.

Alan was not unduly worried about his shoulder, and very enthusiastic to begin his professional career proper. He had been selected to play in a reserve game the day after his operation, and he approached Dr Pearce to see if there was any chance that he might be able to play. The doctor did not examine the wound but said that he was sure that it would be alright to play.

Naturally Alan did so, keeping his well-padded shoulder as much out of harm's way as possible. He was constantly aware of the problem with his shoulder and did not play well.

After three days Dr Pearce re-examined the wound which was found to be weeping, and a powder was applied before re-dressing. From that point fresh dressings were applied daily because of excessive discharge. After about two weeks Dr Pearce removed the stitches, and was adamant that it would heal. Alan was by now very worried because the wound was very painful and seemed to have become larger still. It was not until one month after the operation that Alan was referred to the plastic surgeon, Mr Gavins. At this point the scar was 4 inches by 2 inches.

Because Alan was now so worried about his scar, and no longer felt confident enough to play ice-hockey Mr Gavins agreed to re-excise the wound and close the skin margins again. This did not turn out to improve the scar, if anything it became a little bigger.

After six months Mersey Falcons decided not to renew their option on Alan's contract. He had been able to play several more reserve games but during the six months did not progress sufficiently quickly to the First Team. Alan could not find any other professional club interested in him. He feels that this unhappy outcome could be traced directly to the operation performed by Dr Pearce. In Alan's opinion if it had not been for Dr Pearce he would now be playing professional ice-hockey for Mersey Falcons.

Consequently he approached Mr Brooks who agreed to take on the case. After applying to the courts for access to Alan's medical records Mr Brooks wrote to Mr Gavins and to Professor Peterson in order to gain expert opinions about Dr Pearce's treatment of Alan.

Alan Smith comments

I feel really angry about how I've been treated by Dr Pearce and Mersey Falcons. I know I was good enough. I'm still good enough but I'm 22 now, Falcons turned me out, and all I can do is play my best in the County League and hope that someone else spots me. The thing is it should never have happened. I was alright but the doctor said it would be okay, that I shouldn't have anything get in the way of my career. He said you never know, it might go the wrong way later.

My Mum said it was a disgrace. She was really angry at the time—still is—about the bodge. She said that he was wrong to put in so many stitches, and she could see that it was pulling. Mr Gavins was okay, he seemed to know more about what

continued on next page

continued

he was doing, but after he'd finished it wasn't any better. At the time I just didn't know that there might be this problem. Its a big scar, it itches a lot in the sunshine, and it makes me tense and embarrassed when people look at it. The lads on the building site are right behind me. They think I've been hard done by. Mr Brooks thinks I'll win a few thousand compensation, but how the hell can you compensate me for losing my career?

Dr Pearce's thoughts

I've never been sued before, not in 27 years of general practice, and I've performed a few minor ops like this. I'm insured so I won't have to pay out any money to Smith, but it isn't going to help my reputation at the Falcons. I know that several of the players are on his side.

I accept that perhaps I shouldn't have operated on him. He is very heavily built and has a lot of muscle around his shoulder, and the original scar was over a bony prominence. But he did consent and it is common knowledge that there are risks with any medical procedure.

I'm very worried about my future at the club, but I don't know what I can do about it now. I suppose I can sit it out and hope that Smith can't afford to carry on, or that he can't get any witnesses, or that the judge doesn't think that I was negligent. Or I can do as a couple of colleagues have suggested and talk to Smith, apologise and offer him a couple of thousand as a pay off. I'm not sure but I'll have to make my mind up soon.

Mr Brooks' view

Basically doctors make me sick. I'm quite a devotee of Ian Kennedy. He put the profession firmly in its place—doctors are far too arrogant and too powerful, and they constantly interfere in areas that are not within their competence. The public needs lawyers, and the law, for basic protection. If we weren't an option people like Alan Smith would have to suffer without any hope of redress.

There is absolutely no doubt in my mind that Dr Pearce was negligent. At the very least he should have referred Alan to a plastic surgeon, someone who specialises in this sort of operation. My problem, in fact the only problem I have in this case, is to find other doctors who are prepared to testify that Dr Pearce did not conform to a reasonable medical standard of care. But even though this is such an obvious case of negligence I am not at all confident of finding anybody. I think it is a disgrace. Alan should have enjoyed ten years as a league player, and he's working as a hod carrier—when he can get the work.

Dr Gavins

Dear Mr Brooks,

I am of the opinion that Dr Pearce's handiwork cannot be described as entirely satisfactory, but I do not believe that he was negligent. It is inevitable that removing an ellipse of skin from a site such as this will result in wound tension.

I agreed to re-excise the granulated area in the centre and to re-approximate the skin margins,

continued on next page

continued

in the hope that this would give a somewhat better scar than leaving it alone. I am sorry to say that this was not the result.

I am sorry that I cannot be of any further help to you.

Yours sincerely,

Peter Gavins
Consultant Surgeon

Professor Peterson

Dear Mr Brooks,

re: *Proposed litigation between Alan Smith and Dr Andrew Pearce*

Thank you for your letter of the 10th of this month. I have studied the documents carefully and I am afraid that I can be of little help to you. It is unfortunate that Mr Smith now has a keloid scar of such a size, but this must always be a risk when operating on such a well-built person over a taut area. As far as I can ascertain Dr Pearce acted quite properly throughout the course of treatment. He examined, operated and dressed the wound conscientiously, and when he considered it necessary he arranged for Mr Smith to consult a respected plastic surgeon.

At present Mr Smith's scar is an irritation to him but it is likely that it will reduce in both size and sensitivity, and that eventually he will hardly be aware of its presence. It seems to me that the nub of this case is that Mr Smith's nascent ice-hockey career was unnecessarily handicapped by his shoulder problem, but I cannot see how this can ever be established. As I understand it in order to prove negligence it is not only necessary to establish that a doctor fell below the standard of reasonable medical care, but also that what he did actually caused the alleged suffering. I do not have enough evidence to make a judgement about Dr Pearce's medical competence in this situation, and I suspect that you will be unable to proffer sufficient evidence about cause and effect of the operation on Mr Smith's career, although clearly you may have more expert witnesses than I on this count.

Yours sincerely,

Professor Ian Peterson, FRCGP

Role play/thought play

It is at this point that the role play—either in a group or in the reader's imagination—should take place. What is each of the main characters to do now?

For Alan

He can continue to pursue the claim, or he can drop it at this point. He is not entitled to legal aid, and the case has already cost him over £1000. Solicitors are not cheap, and Professor Peterson's advice cost £250. Alan Smith is not a rich man and cannot call on his parents for help because they too are poor. How much is it worth to him to continue with the case? What satisfaction does he want? What sort of compensation does he expect? What price is he prepared to pay for it?

continued on next page

continued

For Dr Pearce

He has to decide whether to apologise openly to Alan, or to keep quiet and hope that Alan decides to drop the case, or is forced to drop the case through lack of expert support or lack of money. What goes through his mind as he thinks about what to do for the best?

For Mr Brooks

He has competing interests. He wishes to help Alan gain compensation for what Mr Brooks regards as clear medical negligence—incompetence in fact. Also he finds that he likes Alan. Mr Brooks is in business and naturally hopes that the case will go to court, and be successful, to earn him more money. In addition Mr Brooks has a dislike, which is perhaps not entirely based on evidence and reason, of the medical profession. He would be pleased to succeed in a claim for negligence against Dr Pearce.

Mr Brooks knows Alan's financial circumstances. How does he play the situation? How does he deal with any emotional commitment he might feel?

For Mr Gavins

Does he write another letter? Does he try to forestall any litigation against himself? It is not denied that the scar became worse still after his intervention.

Professor Peterson has no further involvement in this case.

What happened?

Alan asked Mr Brooks to continue with the case despite the discouraging responses of the two doctors. He resolved to invest a further £1000 in the search for justice, but he decided that he could not afford to spend more than this. The solicitor wrote to five other professors of general practice for further expert opinion. Three did not reply. Of the two that did one wrote that 'in my opinion Dr Pearce was unwise to operate as he did in the prevailing circumstances. I believe that Dr Pearce's actions are not, and should not be, commonplace amongst general practitioners.' The other wrote in terms which were even more to Alan and his solicitor's liking:

'The swelling was not troublesome, had been accepted by the patient, and represented no sort of hazard to his career in ice-hockey. Given the pathology of post BCG swellings, the presence of keloid in the scar, the site over a bony prominence and the muscular build of the patient, the decision to operate was in my view highly questionable. A prudent general practitioner would have sought specialist advice or taken no action.'

This Professor pledged to testify to this effect in court if necessary.

This expert testimony was sufficient for Mr Brooks to proceed with the claim in negligence. After three further years the case was presented in the High Court. The judges applied the 'Bolam Test' to the claim.

In Alan Smith's case the judges accepted the opinion of the Professor who argued that a 'reasonable' or 'prudent' GP would not have done as Dr Pearce did. They could have chosen to accept other evidence, which was made available to them by the defence, but they held the right to be the ultimate arbiters in this case.

After reading Part II you may wish to re-analyse this case in terms of the doctor's position within the Rings of Uncertainty prior to the operation.

Chapter Three

Man-made Disease?
Man-made Health?

In this chapter further evidence is offered to reinforce the foundations of an argument to come. It is to be asserted that because norms are selected and cannot have an existence wholly independent of human judgement, medicine should rethink its priorities. If it is the case that even where disease is concerned there is no absolute objectivity, then human judgement about human priorities becomes infinitely more important than any imagined impetus to fight disease as something absolutely objectively evil. Almost universal consensus exists that medicine ought to be essentially concerned to combat disease. But what if this consensus can be shown to be mistaken? What if it can be demonstrated that it is not disease, but something else which logically ought to be acknowledged to be the fundamental drive behind medical work?

In Chapters One and Two it was clearly established that when objects, events, activities or people are described as 'normal' or 'abnormal' the description does not somehow simply 'spring from nature'. Normality does not exist as an objective fact. In order for something to become normal or abnormal it has to be said to be so. Normality must emanate in part from a subjective source. Given this, it is a logical step then to say that the same is true of 'disease'. Just as 'normality' must be partially created by a human decision, so 'disease' comes fully into being only on being defined. Although the physical entities and physiological states which are called 'diseases' (for example, bacteria, tumours, sclerosis) actually exist physically, the decision to label them comes from human beings. Microorganisms cause pneumonia. The decision to call a lung 'infected' with them a 'diseased lung' comes entirely from *Homo sapiens*.

For people accustomed to working with diseases thought of as concrete things—as objective entities in their own right—this can be a difficult point to accept. By way of further elucidation consider the following quote from a medical doctor:

> 'All medical science studies facets of behaviour (*by this the author means behaviour in the widest sense, as in either the behaviour of a molecule, an organ of the body, or of a person*) under a wide variety of conditions. Many of these variations we call disease. But the grounds for calling them disease are not any essential part of the studies. Disease is an arbitrary designation.
>
> As illustrating the confusion surrounding the notion of disease, I recall a very precise young physician who asked me what our laboratory considered the normal haemoglobin level of the blood . . . When I answered, "Twelve to sixteen grams, more or less," he was very puzzled. Most laboratories, he pointed out, called 15 grams normal, or perhaps 14.5. He wanted to know how, if my norm was so broad and vague, he could

possibly tell whether a patient suffered from anaemia, or how much anaemia. I agreed that he had quite a problem on his hands, and that it is a very difficult thing to tell. So difficult, in fact, that trying to be too precise is actually misleading, inaccurate, stultifying to thought, and philosophically very unsound.

He wanted to know why I didn't take one hundred or so normal individuals, determine their haemoglobin by our method, and use the resulting figure as the normal value for our method . . . But how are we to pick out the normals? The obvious answer is, just take one or two hundred healthy people, free of disease . . . But that is exactly the difficulty . . . This is travelling in circles. . . .' [43]

A Weed or a Flower—Disease or Health?

What is a weed? The simple answer is that a weed is a plant that is not required. For instance, a dandelion or a daisy in a well-tended lawn. But there is not a plant in the world which can be said objectively to be a weed. Plants become weeds as we call them weeds. The dandelion is not a weed in France where it is often wanted and cultivated for use in salads, and the daisy is not a weed but a flower in a garden where children love to make daisy chains. There are plants, they exist. Some are cultivated and encouraged, but all that *is* objectively—free from human judgement about their value—are different things which we call plants.

What is a weed for one person can be a flower for another. Even for the same labeller, dependent upon the context, a plant can be both a weed and a flower. The 'self-sown' ring of foxgloves around your pond in the front garden can be plants to be cherished, their flowering anticipated with pleasure, whilst that patch of young 'self-sown' foxgloves that has appeared amongst the peas in your vegetable patch are irritating and need to be hoed to death as soon as possible.

As with weeds and flowers, equally with disease and health. There are bodies in various states of growth and decay, some of these states are desirable and others are not. As with plants, what counts as undesirable in one case may be wanted in another. Pneumonia in an otherwise active 20 year old is undesirable. In such a case it seems appropriate to say that the young man is suffering from a disease. But pneumonia in a 91-year-old woman who has recently had a severe stroke might be welcomed by her and her carers—can it be legitimate to define something which brings an easier death a disease? In clinical terms the pneumonia must still be called 'disease', but is such a definition really appropriate, or is this the result of convention only? (Just as some people persist in calling dandelions weeds whilst feeding heaps of them to their tortoises.)

There are many examples of the ambiguity of the 'disease' label. It is not difficult to imagine how a kidney infection in severely incapacitated, terminally ill people might be regarded as more akin to a flower than a weed—at least by those who make the guess that death is better than some types of being alive. Before the industrial revolution moths with black markings on their white wings were said to be victims of a genetic disease because they could be seen clearly on trees and so were easy targets for birds. However, with the soot and grime produced by emerging industry these black markings became advantageous to moths by acting as camouflage. In certain contexts 'disease' can clearly be desirable to the person who is said to have it. For instance, social scientists describe certain people as having adopted 'the sick role'.

For those who take on 'the sick role' the disease grants them certain privileges—usually they are excused their work responsibilities, and often they are looked after by others. It is not uncommon for people, on hearing that so-and-so has a cold and has a week of sick leave, to reflect on their own work pressures and stresses and to wish quickly and genuinely that they had a cold too!

Perhaps the most obvious example where 'disease' is desirable is that of vaccination. When people are immunised they are deliberately infected with a small dose of an attenuated virus in order that their bodies build up immunity to infection, thus at least minimising their suffering if they happen to contract a larger dose in the future. Whatever the ultimate justification in terms of disease avoidance, it cannot be denied that the initial 'disease' is wanted. Surely this calls the labelling into question.

> 'The blight that strikes at corn or at potatoes is a human invention for if man wished to cultivate parasites (rather than potatoes or corn) there would be no 'blight', but simply the necessary foddering of the parasite-crop . . . Outside the significances that man voluntarily attaches to certain conditions, *there are no illnesses or diseases in nature*. We are nowadays so heavily indoctrinated with deriving from the technical medical discoveries of the last century and a half that we are tempted to think that nature does contain diseases. Just as the sophisticated New Yorker classes the excrement of dogs and cats as one more form of "pollution" ruining the pre-established harmony of pavements and gardens, so does modern technologised man perceive nature to be mined and infested with all kinds of specifically morbid entities and agencies. What, he will protest, are there no diseases in nature? Are there not infectious and contagious bacilli? Are there not definite and objective lesions in the cellular structures of the human body? Are there not fractures of bones, the fatal ruptures of tissues, the malignant multiplications of tumorous growths? Are not these, surely, events of nature? Yet these, as natural events, do not—prior to the human social meanings we attach to them—constitute illnesses, sicknesses, or diseases. The fracture of the septuagenarian's femur has, within the world of nature, no more significance than the snapping of an autumn leaf from its twig: and the invasion of the human organism by cholera germs carries with it no more the stamp of 'illness' than does the souring of milk by other forms of bacteria.' [44]

Presumably without intending it, in this paper written in the early 1970s Sedgewick provides a perfect example of his own point. He writes:

> '. . . the example of tooth-decay is suggestive: among millions of British working class families, it is taken for granted that children will lose their teeth and require artificial dentures. The process of tooth loss is not seen as a disease, but as something like an act of fate.' [45]

Here Sedgewick is reinforcing the point that tooth loss is so common that we choose not to label it as a disease process, but think of it as natural. It follows that—if we chose to—we could redesignate tooth loss, and—by fiat—it would become disease.

This change—this *'normality shift'*—actually seems to have happened. Nowadays standards have changed, dental care has progressed, fewer holes are made in teeth in order to cut out minor decay, and the presence of fluoride in the general water supply and in toothpaste is said to have greatly reduced the incidence of decay [46]. In the 1990s the working-class child who will need to have dentures—ever in his lifetime—is in the minority and will almost certainly be defined as suffering from, or as having suffered from, disease. Whether it is said that changes in standards of dental care have changed the reality of disease, or merely that the system of classification has changed, it must be concluded that the status of disease is less than objective in this example.

Why it can be useful to call some states of existence 'diseased'

The above analysis is not meant to imply that it is entirely wrong to describe certain human conditions as 'diseased' or that it is pointless. On the contrary, disease ascriptions are important in medicine because:

(1)   To describe certain clinical states as 'diseases' and others as not makes possible both diagnosis and prognosis: labelling is part of the attempt to predict outcome. From the point of view of clinical medicine 'disease' is a term used to indicate a deviation from *accepted* norms. Disease and abnormality are intrinsically linked. Symptoms and signs of disease are commonly found to recur in constant patterns, which are in turn called 'syndromes' or 'symptom-complexes'. 'Disease' and its associated labels help doctors pinpoint specific ailments and prescribe appropriate treatment—obviously it is not enough to say "Peter has a problem with his throat" when he has "tonsillitis" and not "laryngitis".

(2)   Labelling allows meaningful communication in medicine—the existence of the terminology of disease provides taxonomy and a technical language, both of which are necessary for doctors to understand each other and to undertake shared research.

Why it can be disadvantageous to label some states of existence as 'diseased'

A central problem now commonly associated with labelling certain states of being as 'diseased' and others as 'healthy' is that to classify a condition as a disease can have the effect of legitimising intervention by doctors in areas of a person's life which seem to be beyond the remit of clinical science. For many thinkers, medicine, by defining certain states as disease, assumes an exclusive expert role in 'curing' these states even if the people who are 'diseased' do not want the 'cures' which medicine offers. But medicine persists, nevertheless, operating with a simple view that since diseases are—by definition—bad they ought to be eliminated. There are countless articles in the literature of medical sociology and medical ethics critical of such 'medical imperialism'. For instance Englehardt and colleagues have written:

'Labelling a condition or state as a disease has had, and continues to have, serious political, economic, and social consequences. If a particular behaviour or problem is approached as a matter of health and disease, the medical profession is thereby conceptually licensed to diagnose, treat, and otherwise intervene.

It is thus no small matter to the person who uses drugs or who engages in various forms of sexual activity whether such behaviour is viewed as indicative of disease, criminality, taste, or immorality. Liability and responsibility are often waived when a physiological condition is labelled as a disease or illness, often to be replaced by involuntary treatment, institutional confinement, and surgical or pharmacological manipulation.

. . . medicine has often deemed it appropriate to classify various sexual activities, habits, and ethnic differences as diseases. The importation of biases and prejudices into medical classifications of disease has had disastrous consequences for various social groups. The danger that subjective preferences and tastes can masquerade as objective scientific judgements is a danger requiring vigilant and critical conceptual attention.

. . . Decisions about whether a condition or behaviour is best conceived of as a disease or as indicative of health are not made in a social vacuum. As social conditions change, persons who once struggled to establish certain behaviours, for example, homosexuality, heroin addiction, gambling, or alcoholism, as diseases may find themselves arguing that such states ought not to be so classified. The history of the medical profession's activities regarding sensitive areas of personal behaviour and life-style should give the reader pause as to whether current medical attitudes toward disease reflect an uncritical acceptance of views based only upon tradition, and the extent to which the concepts of health and disease are conceptually independent from moral and value choices and justifications.' [47]

Medicine's Category Mistake

Many readers may have found the developing argument increasingly bizarre. Indeed it may appear that everything that has been said so far has been destructive, so consistently negative that the point of collapse is close. In fact, quite the opposite is true. The aim of the exercise so far has been to remove unjustified assumptions and presumptions; not to undermine medicine, not as a playful diversion in philosophical scepticism, but as a necessary stage in a programme of construction. Every builder knows that land has to be cleared, and sometimes existing buildings have to be demolished, before relevant, modern structures can be erected. Equally it is not uncommon for the best parts of demolished buildings to be incorporated into the new ones.

Medicine seems to have arrived at a point where it is trapped by both semantics and social convention. Unquestionably the majority of doctors wish to care for people, wish to assist them 'back to health'. Or if this is not possible, wish at least to ensure that they do not suffer more than they have to. The notion that *disease is the enemy of medicine* is so deeply ingrained within medical literature, and in the minds of the world's populations, that it is scarcely credible to suggest that medicine reassess its purpose, that medicine might shift its orientation. But unless it does so the discipline is condemned by tradition to try to prevent or cure *whatever* a particular time or society defines as a disease. And since it can be clearly demonstrated that there is an element of choice in the naming of disease, doctors will continue to be accused of being agents of social control. Inevitably, many doctors will be social controllers—compelled to be so by the expectations of language and society—even though this is not the chosen role, not the *raison d'être* of that particular doctor.

In order to see a way out of this state of affairs, which many doctors find unsatisfactory, it is necessary to take two further steps. These moves develop the argument of this book. They are:

(1)   To take a lead from a philosopher of mind who invented the notion of the 'category mistake'. This notion can offer an important insight. It highlights a way for doctors to begin to accept the possibility that medicine has gone too far along a path that is too narrow.

(2)   To consider an expanded rationale for medicine, a rationale of 'work for health' rather than 'work against disease'. This alternative theoretical basis for medical activity can *liberate medicine* from the restrictions of semantics and convention, from the misdirection of the narrow path. In addition, this alternative has many implications for health care as a whole—some of which are outlined in the closing pages of this book.

Applying a philosophical insight

Gilbert Ryle, an Oxford Professor of Philosophy, introduced the idea of a 'category mistake'. By this he was referring to the mistake that people sometimes make when they try to represent facts that properly belong in a particular category as if they belong in a different one. In his book, Ryle was concerned to explain a particular 'category mistake', which he believes many philosophers have made, following the notable example of Descartes. This mistake is to talk about 'mental events'—thought processes such as believing, regretting, or hoping—as if they are things of a quite different nature to other human processes. In this way a dichotomy is invented rather than discovered: a myth comes into being that moving, eating and breathing belong to one category while thinking belongs to quite another. The former processes are part of the mechanical body, while the latter process is part of something non-mechanical and non-spatial—something which we call *mind*.

Ryle illustrates the general idea of a 'category mistake' with a number of examples, of which these are two:

> 'A foreigner visiting Oxford or Cambridge for the first time is shown a number of colleges, libraries, playing fields, museums, scientific departments and administrative offices. He then asks 'But where is the University? I have seen where the members of the Colleges live, where the Registrar works, where the scientists experiment and the rest. But I have not yet seen the University in which reside and work the members of your University.' It has then to be explained to him that the University is not another collateral institution, some ulterior counterpart to the colleges, laboratories and offices which he has seen. The University is just the way in which all that he has already seen is organized. When they are seen and when their co-ordination is understood, the University has been seen. His mistake lay in his innocent assumption that it was correct to speak of Christ Church, the Bodleian Library, the Ashmolean Museum *and* the University, to speak, that is, as if 'the University' stood for an extra member of the class of which these other units are members. He was mistakenly allocating the University to the same category as that to which the other institutions belong.

A foreigner watching his first game of cricket learns what are the functic
bowlers, the batsmen, the fielders, the umpires and the scorers. He then
there is no one left on the field to contribute the famous element of team-spirit. I see
who does the bowling, the batting and the wicket-keeping; but I do not see whose role
it is to exercise *esprit de corps*." Once more, it would have to be explained that he was
looking for the wrong type of thing. Team-spirit is not another cricketing operation
supplementary to all of the other special tasks. It is, roughly, the keenness with which
each of the special tasks is performed, and performing a task keenly is not performing
two tasks. Certainly exhibiting team-spirit is not the same thing as bowling or catching,
but nor is it a third thing such that we can say that the bowler first bowls *and* then
exhibits team-spirit or that a fielder is at a given moment *either* catching *or* displaying
esprit de corps.

These illustrations of category-mistakes have a common feature which must be noticed.
The mistakes were made by people who did not know how to wield the concepts
University . . . and *team-spirit*. Their puzzles arose from inability to use certain terms
in the English vocabulary.' [48]

What Ryle is attempting to show in his book is that those philosophers who think
of 'mind' as being something logically different from 'body' have committed a 'category
mistake'. They are looking for the wrong type of thing. To avoid the mistake they
should think of mind in the correct category. It would be better to regard 'mind'
like the University in Ryle's first illustration, as 'organisation'—or perhaps like *esprit
de corps*—as arising out of sufficient complexity, just as team-spirit comes into being
given sufficient keenness in the team members.

A pervasive category mistake in medicine   Medicine's conception of the notions
'disease' and 'health' can be thought of as 'category mistakes', although the inverse
of the 'category mistake' made over 'mind' which Ryle suggests. Whereas Ryle is
criticising a tradition in philosophy which regards 'mind' as additional, as *some thing*
else, to 'body', it is possible to criticise medicine for the reverse. *Medicine's 'category
mistake' is to regard 'health' and 'disease' as intimately linked, as if on a continuum,
so that the more disease a person has, the further away from perfect health he is. For
those who make the category mistake, disease and health are always related, one always
depends upon the relative strength or weakness of the other.*

This is to place both health and disease in the same general category when this
is actually a mistake. Instead it is correct to regard these as different categories, albeit
often with significant overlaps. Precisely why health is in a different logical category
to disease takes time to explain. A summary of this complicated explanation is offered
in the section which follows.

Health

In order to understand how it can possibly be said that medicine has committed a
'category mistake' by concentrating on disease when trying to create health, it is
necessary to think through what health means. Two crucial features will emerge from
this analysis: firstly, that work for health can legitimately be undertaken without any
reference to disease and illness, and secondly, that far from this resulting in a
'meaningless concept'—where anything at all can count as health work—clear limits

beyond which actions cannot be described as work for health can be shown. Because it is possible to be so clear about the limits of work for health, this theory is infinitely more precise than work for health thought of exclusively as anti-disease work. Since the notion of health work as anti-disease is so vague and woolly it has been possible for some doctors to attempt to justify anything—from deceit to murder—as proper health work because as a result disease is avoided, lessened or cured.

It is important to recognise at the outset that by arguing that medicine should become *work for health* it is not being suggested that doctors should become social workers or teachers instead of medics—doctors have extensive clinical knowledge and skills which must always be the base for their practice. But it is suggested that because these skills are applied to people, and because judgements which are not essentially clinical must be made in medical work, it is vital—in order that the highest quality interventions are made—that doctors not only learn more about the basis of such judgements (that they are taught some law, social science, and economics, for example), but that they are able to make them within a clear framework for practice which *makes sense* for each doctor, and which has a clear and practical rationale.

A path towards a better understanding of the nature of health

'Health' is a difficult word. At once it seems that we each know intuitively what it means, but also that we are unable to express its meaning in a way that will be universally agreed. Whatever definition of health we hit upon there will always be some legitimate objection to it. And there will be alternative definitions which also seem to be strong candidates for the title *the* definition of health.

A review of the literature on theories and definitions of health reveals that there are a number of well-supported, and sometimes well-argued, theories of health which are in competition with one another. It is not simply that they are battling for *the Crown*, for the right to be generally acknowledged as the best theory. Rather they seem to be attempting to occupy different, or at least partly different, territories. Thus, they are bound to be incompatible. Yet each seems not only to be making sense, but also to be referring to 'something' which many people would recognise as 'what health means'.

Consider these three theories of health as examples. Note how each makes sense, but note also how because of differences in meaning the three simply cannot be combined into a coherent overall theory.

The WHO theory   The theory of the World Health Organization (WHO) that 'Health is a state of complete physical, mental and social well-being and not merely the absence of disease and infirmity.' [49]

The not-ill theory   The theory that a person is healthy if he or she has no disease or illness.

The coping theory   The theory that a person is healthy if he or she has the wherewithal to adapt to problems of life—not just clinical problems.

Each of these theories has its articulate advocates and each will make sense to many, if not most, people.

Competing theories of health

The World Health Organization's view of health, the **WHO theory**, tends to evoke in some people both a future picture and a remembrance of ease and contentment—something which only the most unfortunate human beings never feel at any time in their lives. It sets an ambitious target at which to aim, in the belief that the higher the aim the higher the outcome—even if the stated target is missed. Taken literally, if health is a state of complete physical, mental and social well-being, then a person cannot be healthy if she is diseased or ill. Nor can she be described as healthy if she is unhappy, or bored, or living on her own in a terraced house in Warrington when she wants to be married and living in France.

The **not-ill theory**, the view that a person is healthy if he or she is not suffering from disease or illness, is held (often only implicitly) in some medical circles. Crudely speaking, the argument goes like this: since medicine is health-work, and the proper subject of medical attention and activity is disease and illness, then it follows that the key measure of success in health work must be the extent to which disease and illness have been prevented or eliminated.

As with the WHO theory of health a person cannot be healthy if he is diseased (disregarding the philosophical difficulties over the definition of disease). But the two theories do not share a view about the extent to which the shape of other aspects of a person's life should play a role in the assessment of his health. For the World Health Organization, at the very worst, a person must be fulfilled and productive to be healthy. But on the not-ill theory, provided a person has no problems which can be defined in clinical terms, he must be healthy. Even if a man is friendless and in despair for his future, he can be said to be healthy.

The **coping theory**, that health is essentially an ability to adapt to life's problems, appears at first sight to have much in common with the idealistic dictum of the World Health Organization. But not on closer inspection. For where the World Health Organization insist on wellbeing and fulfilment for health, the coping theory allows a diseased and unfulfilled person the label healthy—so long as she has a personal strength, an ability to shake off knocks, to fight back, and to carry on with living. According to the coping theory, an elderly lady recovering from a hip-replacement operation who contracts a lung infection shortly after hearing of the death of her husband, is none the less healthy if she possesses the physical and emotional strength—the resilience—to recover from all the insults. Equally, a person without a disease who does not have the resources to respond positively whenever trouble—physical or otherwise—strikes ought not to be described as healthy according to this theory. Thus the **coping theory** is incompatible not only with the **WHO theory** but also with the **not-ill theory**.

The disagreement between theories of health is and will be never-ending. The more theories of health that are invented, the more complicated the analysis becomes. As the complexity of the subject grows, so does the realisation that it is impossible to combine the various options into some grand design which will reveal the true story of health. There are simply too many inconsistencies, incompatibilities, and reasonable points of view. But this is not to say that puzzling about the nature of health is pointless. It is possible to make some overall sense of this confusing subject, and then to erect a framework for practical problem-solving on this solid base.

A common factor

Despite the bafflement it *is* possible to identify a factor common to these disparate accounts. Although it is not possible to point to a single, simple, definition of health, a component common to each theory can be identified. This factor is so obvious that it appears trite. But it is actually a significant step forward in the attempt to gain a usable grasp of the nature of health, and so of the moral framework within which doctors might choose to practice.

The common factor that must be present in any legitimate theory of health is this: *any genuine theory of health will be concerned to identify one or more human potentials which might develop, but which are presently or likely to be* **blocked**. *Health work, however it is defined, will seek first to discover and then prevent or remove obstacles to the achievement of human potential.*

Dependent upon the theory of health invoked, the appropriate obstacles for the attention of health workers will vary from only specific clinical conditions (as is the case in the **not-ill theory**) to barriers to free choice, to the development of the imagination, and to personal creativity (as is the case in the theory of health offered later in this chapter). On the former view the only potentials which warrant the attention of health workers will be physiological dysfunction (possibly stretching to include some mental disorders, even if these apparently lack physical cause), while according to the broader theory, ignorance and lack of confidence can be obstacles in the way of the achievement of better health. But however narrowly or broadly defined one's chosen theory of health is, it is *essential that it focuses on obstacles to latent human achievement.* If it does not, then it cannot be a theory of health.

Focusing the category mistake in medicine

It is at this point that the category mistake of medicine can begin to be brought into focus. Disease is an obstacle to desired human growth, and it is correct to say that the fight against this must generally speaking count as health work. However, it is not possible purely to combat disease. Always there will be additional factors which must be taken into account.

In fact it is not possible to treat disease in an entirely pure way. Any imaginable scenario where such a thing might happen will be bizarre. How might a doctor purely treat disease? Perhaps the image which comes nearest is one of the gowned surgeon waiting in the operating theatre, armed with the technology and technique to cut away disease, after which the patient will be wheeled away by others. But even if it were true that such human islands could exist, that a surgeon could always be entirely disinterested in the person under his charge, other doctors would have to be involved in other processes, processes which might be necessary as a result of disease, but which have no effect or bearing on the disease *per se*. For instance, the general practitioner would most likely have to diagnose the disease in the first place, a process which must at least involve communication and interpretation. Some other doctor might then have to convey the need for an operation, naturally a sensitive communication. After this, the patient might also be helped by counselling or other support. He would also have to consent to the operation, and so need to be informed of what is to happen to him, and the main risks involved. Following his operation it would almost certainly be necessary for him to adjust physically and mentally, to convalesce and recuperate. Even when the disease is gone, more help is always required.

However far one might try to stretch the notion of disease it must always be the case that no disease can exist independently of a host. Human beings suffer disease—diseases can only be as a part of a complex and varied entity. In health work the interaction is not undertaken with a disease as a separate thing, but with a person who has the disease (or at least who is said to have a disease). Inevitably other factors are important. For example, how a person feels, what a person wants, and what a person is able to do, both before and after any intervention, cannot be divorced from even the most scientific medical procedure.

The most obvious manifestation of the category mistake is revealed in the following statement: *in order to work for health it is necessary as a priority to defeat disease.* Although this may on occasions be true—for instance where the disease is serious, where there is a successful treatment for it, and where the patient wishes that the treatment be carried out and is willing to risk the possible costs—it is not necessarily always true. For instance, it may be that the disease might be borne if it is not interfering impossibly with the diseased person's life priorities, and where the risks of the treatment seem too great (as Mrs Sidaway argued, see page 33).

However, this is only one part of the category mistake. The manifestation expressed in the above statement could be construed merely as a question of *emphasis,* whereas a category mistake must be radical, not a matter of degree.

In the following section it is demonstrated how the belief that health and disease form a continuum:

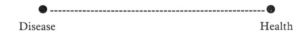

Disease   Health

is mistaken. Instead health and disease should be thought of as *separate categories*

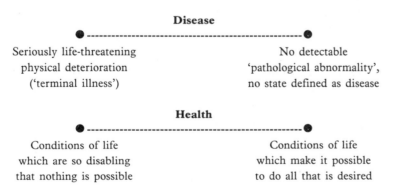

Disease

Seriously life-threatening   No detectable
physical deterioration   'pathological abnormality',
('terminal illness')   no state defined as disease

Health

Conditions of life   Conditions of life
which are so disabling   which make it possible
that nothing is possible   to do all that is desired

Before this distinction can be fully explained it is first necessary to consider a possible objection to the identification of the common factor. This is that to say that 'work for health means work to remove obstacles to human potential' is hopelessly general.

A naive view of health

Characterised as 'set against obstacles to the achievement of biological and chosen potentials', it is true to say that the notion of health outlined so far is general and quite naive. It is a starting point, but it is not sufficiently developed to be of practical use to doctors searching for a clear framework within which to practice. In particular, as it stands it is vulnerable to the following criticisms.

Tinker, tailor, soldier, sailor . . .   Cast in such a general way this view of health appears to make almost everybody a health worker—from teachers and social workers to bakers, policemen and sewage workers. Surely not every person who works towards the removal of obstacles which get in the way, or which may get in the way, of the development of human potential, should be described as a 'health worker'. Only health professionals—primarily only those qualified in medicine and nursing—ought to be known as health workers.

Some potentials are evil . . .   Not all obstacles to human potential ought to be removed. Some obstacles actually ought to be *encouraged* because they can act as blocks to bad, undesirable human potentials. It is not sufficient to say that work for health consists in preventing or eliminating any obstacles to human achievement, since this accommodates too much—it is far better to cast work for health in narrower terms: for instance, in terms of effort against disease and illness. This offers precision and the reassurance that the obstacles of disease and illness ought not to be encouraged. Without specifics health workers might at times be cast in the ludicrous role of working to enable evil, stupidity, or even disease (since disease is one of an indefinite number of human potentials). A theory of health which cannot come up with some workable way of differentiating between potentials worth developing and those not worth having is practically useless.

Where should I begin to work for health . . . ?   Human potential is whatever a human being might become. Almost anything in the world might be an obstacle to one of these potentials. If this is the extent of the precision of the definition 'work for health', then doctors face an impossible task in deciding upon their priorities. How does a doctor working for health in such a broad way decide where to begin?

It is possible to meet each of these criticisms. In order to do so it is necessary to put forward a more complete theory of health.

Developing a firmer view of health

Fortunately it is possible to develop a more precise, and more useful, view of health.

Consider this extract from an earlier work:

'Work for health is concerned with enabling fulfilling achievements. It aims for the achievement of normative or positive potentials. Medicine is an example of a means which is employed to help people achieve norms. For instance, it is accepted that "normal bodies" and "normal children" will develop in certain predictable ways, such is their normative potential. If they are developing abnormally, then steps might be taken to attempt to bring them nearer to a normal state, unless they are regarded as exceptional bodies.

Ideas about 'positive potentials' will vary, but what is common to the notion of positive potential is that individuals will seek to achieve a range of states which they believe will enhance their lives in a variety of ways. For instance, people might aim to improve physically—by exercising, by dieting, by cosmetic surgery, by other surgery—or intellectually—by reading and taking courses of education—or socially, or emotionally. Not all people will see these goals as positive, but (each) will recognise personally enhancing potentials and set about fulfilling them.

The idea of 'positive potential' can be contrasted with the idea of *liability*. Liabilities are the sorts of problem which act against the achievement of positive or normative potential. For instance, disease is a liability which, if circumstances had been different need not have occurred. Ignorance is a liability which, if not overcome, can prevent the achievement of all sorts of positive potential. Negative potentials are liabilities.

It is possible to strip this distinction of at least some of its ambiguity. Work for health is work which aims to enable and to enhance by providing foundations for the achievement of potentials. It is opposed to liabilities because they are debilitating. The distinction hinges on the difference between the ideas of *enhancing* and *debilitating*.

Work for health will be concerned with encouraging normative and positive potentials because these potentials have the effect of opening up possibilities for achieving more potentials, whereas negative potentials reduce the number of possible potentials.' [50]

Basically, what this extract argues is that good health care (and so good medicine) will first determine an acceptable range of normality. It will say 'these states are normal'—and by implication desirable—and these abnormal.

Good medicine will then work to prevent or cure abnormality. But on top of this it will be both possible and desirable, in most people's cases, to work to enable other potentials to flourish regardless of the presence or absence of a clinical condition. For instance, in addition to any medical treatment deemed necessary, it might be possible to help a mentally handicapped child play a musical instrument, or to help a harassed mother find better ways of educating or entertaining her three young children. Such possibilities can be called *positive potentials*. Work to bring them into existence should be thought of as work for health.

Normative and positive potentials can be distinguished from *liabilities*, such as disease and ignorance. Health work should seek ultimately to generate only *enhancing* potentials—only those potentials which open up more possibilities for fulfilled existence—or at least leave the number of possibilities at their present level. According to every theory of health, it is a simple contradiction to say that health work should seek to create *situations which diminish overall*—states which reduce the possibilities open to a person.

Dwarfing

The idea of *liability* can be translated into the more memorable notion of *dwarfing**. Work for health has been described in this way:

*This label is not intended to cause offence.

'Work for health is work directed against the intentional or accidental dwarfing of people. Since every aspect of a person's being can be dwarfed, work for health should be correspondingly comprehensive.' [51]

This quote focuses attention on the notion of *liability*. Liabilities both exist and have the potential to exist—they are possible ways of being. Liabilities limit a person, closing down opportunities for desirable development. *Dwarfing* is a term which describes the process whereby liabilities—the limiting of options—are brought into being. As such, dwarfing can be thought of as the direct opposite of work for health. For example, if a person is not told the truth about her clinical condition, then she is obviously deceived. Whatever the motive for the deception, however beneficial the outcome is thought to be for the patient or her family and friends, she is nevertheless deliberately dwarfed. She might have understood more about her life, but she has been denied this opportunity. The only possible justification for this dwarfing, or any other dwarfing, will be that the policy avoids worse dwarfing. However, where the dwarfing involves a decrease in what might be understood by a person, then the justification must demonstrate how the person's future understanding will be expanded (this point is explained more fully in Chapter Six).

To give less controversial examples, if a person suffers avoidable damage as the result of a doctor's negligence (see page 31) then he can be said to have been dwarfed in proportion to the extent of the damage which might not have been. And further, if a person is prescribed a drug (say, a tranquilliser such as Valium) and she becomes habituated, then she loses a degree of control over her life. In this way she is dwarfed: a potential she had which might have enhanced her life (or at least which would count as a normative potential) has been lost, and replaced by a liability. Whether or not this dwarfing can be justified depends upon: (a) whether the loss of control due to stress or depression was greater than the habituation; *and* (b) whether there were other, less risky, ways of solving the original problem—ways that would not endanger her welfare or her choice. Only if the answer to (a) is 'yes' and (b) is 'no', will the dwarfing have a chance of standing up to examination.

In some circumstances dwarfings are unavoidable. These are usually the hardest cases in which to reach a decision, the cases where moral balancing—a weighing of the theoretical and practical factors—is necessary. However, the presence of the category mistake in medicine means that currently some avoidable dwarfings are implemented when they ought not to be. Good intentions are sometimes polluted by an underestimation of the richness of the notion of health care.

Priorities

The distinction between *enhancement* and *dwarfing* can help to clarify which potentials to work on in the case of specific individuals. The worth of this clarification can be recognised as soon as the idea is applied to a person in real life. But it does not help doctors decide on general priorities, nor does it offer a rationale for choosing to enable one form of development in an individual, and not another form—or for choosing one dwarfing over another when some dwarfing is inevitable.

What might general priorities for work for health broadly conceived look like? The following suggestions were made in an earlier book [52]. They remain central:

'Some of the foundations which make up health are of the highest importance for all people. These are:

(1) The basic needs of food, drink, shelter, warmth, and purpose in life.
(2) Access to the widest possible information about all factors which have an influence on a person's life.
(3) The skill and confidence to assimilate this information. In most societies literacy and numeracy are needed in older children and adults. People need to be able to understand how the information applies to them, and to be able to make reasoned decisions about what action to take in the light of their information.
(4)   The recognition that an individual is never totally isolated from other people and the external world. People are complex wholes who cannot be fully understood separated from the influence of their environment, which is itself a whole of which they are a part. People are not like marbles packed in boxes, where they are a community only because of their forced proximity. People are part of their whole surroundings, like cells in a single body. This fact compels the recognition that a person should not strive to fulfil personal potentials which will undermine the basic foundations for achievement of other people. In short, an essential condition for health in human beings who are aware of the implications of their actions is that they have an awareness of a basic duty they have because they are people in a community.

Other foundations for achievement are bound to vary between individuals dependent upon which potentials can realistically be achieved. For instance, a diseased person, a person in a damp and dilapidated house, a person in prison, a fit young athlete, a terminal patient, and an expectant mother all need the central conditions which constitute part of their healths, but in addition they require other specific foundations in order to enable them to make the most of their present lives.' [53]

These central conditions can be pictured as *foundations*, or as a set of conditions for living. The central conditions can be thought of as a stage on which a person might achieve what is possible for her.

'A person's optimum state of health is equivalent to the state of the set of conditions which fulfil or enable a person to work to fulfil his or her realistic chosen and biological potentials. Some of these conditions are of the highest importance for all people. Others are variable dependent upon individual abilities and circumstances.

The actual degree of health that a person has at a particular time depends upon the degree to which these conditions are realised in practice.' [54]

Precisely what does this statement about the nature of health mean? The radical nature of this theory of health, both in a practical and philosophical sense, seems not yet to have been fully appreciated.

Study it carefully. Implicit within the statement is the opinion that a person's health should not be thought of as an absolute. Nor should a person have to possess ideal wellbeing in order to have health. It is quite different from the wild optimism which lies behind the WHO theory. In contrast to the other theories of health it is argued that it is most accurate and practical to see health as a stage, made up of a number of different movable building blocks, upon which a person must perform: a platform upon which she must live—upon which she has to construct her happiness and her success, and bear her failures. If some of these building blocks are missing then a person may still be able to move on the stage, but to a lesser extent than she otherwise might. In just the same way, if part of the stage owned by a school were found to be rotten and in need of repair a day before a play is to be performed, the show would go on even though some parts of the play might have to be cut. Just because a person has become limited in what she can do does not necessarily mean that she is now completely unhealthy, nor does the fact that she has less health than she did necessarily legitimise medical intervention.

The above statement claims, quite deliberately, that a person's health should be thought of as *equivalent* to the state of the platform on which she might achieve. The term 'health' thought of in this way is not used to describe only the internal state of the person—the shape his body and his mind is in. Nor is it intended that the existence of the stage should *depend* upon 'the absence of disease' to glue it together. The presence or absence of a disease may not be the primary consideration, and in some cases need not be a consideration at all in the assessment of a person's state of health.

This theory of health claims that a person's health can be thought of in a sense wider than the properties of the individual herself. This conclusion is far from absurd. In fact it is the only fully coherent conclusion which can be drawn once it is accepted that work for health is work to enable people to do more than they would otherwise be able to do. The secret to understanding the nature of health as *foundations* is to recognise its necessary relationship with autonomy, with the extent to which a person is free to act in his life. Once this is recognised (and this link is argued for extensively in the pages that are to come) then there can be only an arbitrary distinction between work focused on factors internal to a person, and work focused on factors external to him.

Critics might argue that this takes work for health far beyond the medical. This point is quite correct. Critics might claim further that this renders the assessment of a person's health impossible since account would have to be taken of every single factor which affects what a person can do—from whether or not she has a cold, to whether she is loved and has any money. This point is also partly correct—to achieve a fully accurate measure of the state of a person's health involves so many disparate factors that it probably cannot be done [55]. However, it is possible to gain a general grasp, and often fairly easy to decide upon the factors of a person's life which need the most urgent attention.

Finally, critics might claim that to believe that a person's health can change solely as the result of external factors is simply ridiculous. If this is to be the case then as a person is rehoused, or as she takes a well-earned holiday, or as she feels happy to have the sun on her face, then her health changes. Surely, health should not be thought of in this way. In fact there is no reason why it should not be thought of like this, so long as it is possible to understand the practical implications of the theory, and so long as it remains possible to say '*this is legitimate health work, that is not*'. Both these conditions are quite possible. The theory that health is *equivalent* to the set of conditions which permit a person *to do* results in no more absurdity than the theory that a person becomes unhealthy only when she contracts a disease. Firstly, just as a judgement must be made about which are the conditions of life most relevant to the assessment of a person's health, so the designation of a state as a disease involves a judgement. There needs to be a decision, for instance about which bacteria cause diseases (and under which circumstances), and which do not. Secondly, if it is a problem for the theory that *health is equivalent to the conditions which allow doing*, in that the adoption of this theory implies that a person's state of health is constantly in flux—changing in status from one moment to the next—then exactly the same applies to the so-called simpler theory. As a cold runs its course a person's state of health must fluctuate according to the symptoms and the level of infection. As a person becomes depressed during the day her 'health status' is constantly moving even on the 'health as the absence of disease' theory. As a person recovers from a road traffic accident he steadily 'gets better'—his 'health' improves bit by bit as he convalesces. In just the same way, on the broader theory, his health can be affected bit by bit by the amount of external support he receives, by the friends that continue to come to see him, by the news that his boss has held his job open for him. It is not that these things have an *affect* on his 'internal health status'; no, they are themselves *part of* his health status.

Naturally, work for health thought of in this way becomes extensive, but the best health carers know this anyway, and work implicitly according to some sort of unarticulated broad theory. On this view medical care becomes only a part of a broader endeavour of work for health, not essential to it. The decisions of governments about what are to count as acceptable minimum standards of welfare for their people can have a far greater role, for better or worse, in affecting the health of societies.

According to the theory that health is the foundation for achievement, it is best to think of health in this way (Figure 3.1).

The numbered blocks are meant to represent the movable sections of a portable stage. The more blocks there are, and the better their condition, the freer a person will be. Through the provision of enabling conditions a person will usually gain personal control over his life. Generally speaking, the better the conditions, the higher the level of control the person will have. If the person can stand upon the four central blocks (the central conditions listed above) in good order, then that person will, by definition, have a high level of health. If, in addition to the solid blocks of the stage, he has no disease and enjoys good social and environmental amenities (both of which are circumstances which might be defined to give content to block five), then his degree of health may be higher still. The task for any true health worker is to recognise the importance of the foundations in practical context—to identify for each individual those which are lacking or those which are in need of most renovation—and to work on the foundations most appropriate to the skills of that health worker. For example, this means that the social worker, whilst being aware of the work that is required on other foundations, might be best advised to concentrate on blocks two and four (the number of each block corresponds with the central conditions outlined above), whilst the medical doctor might be best placed by his special training and skills to focus on blocks three and five (when five is expressed as disease cure), dependent upon what work is considered to be most necessary.

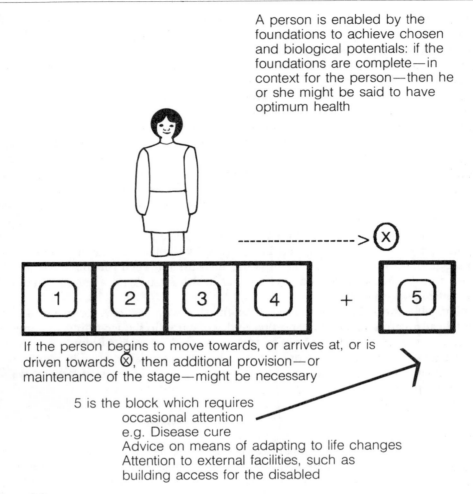

A person is enabled by the foundations to achieve chosen and biological potentials: if the foundations are complete—in context for the person—then he or she might be said to have optimum health

If the person begins to move towards, or arrives at, or is driven towards ⊗, then additional provision—or maintenance of the stage—might be necessary

5 is the block which requires occasional attention e.g. Disease cure Advice on means of adapting to life changes Attention to external facilities, such as building access for the disabled

Figure 3.1

The better the shape of the stage—the more the different sections of the stage are intact (and the more of them that there are)—the better the state of a particular person's health. Health must be viewed realistically, in the context of what is possible for a particular person. A person can be perfectly at liberty within the realm of what is possible for him, even if his stage is not as sound as someone else's. So, if a person has a handicap or an incurable chronic disease which will not disappear naturally, yet has hope, a home, things to do, and friends, then he might be said to have good or even optimum health for him. Health workers must identify the blocks of the stage that it is *realistic* to work on. They must not hope for miracles, nor must they mistakenly, inappropriately, try to work on blocks of the stage which they can never hope to provide, restore, or replace.

The view of health as a platform on which to live, rather than as an idea which encompasses everything there is to a person, carries with it the notion that what a person *does* is not the business of health workers. It is the ability of people to do, or to choose to do, as many things—to take as many paths—as possible that is the essential health concern. Doctors who espouse the theory of health as foundations will accept work for health to mean the creation of autonomy, self-direction, and personal control. They will see that this is the essence of health work, and they will come to see more clearly where they should call a halt.

Review of the Argument of the Book So Far

Up to this stage of the book several arguments have been advanced which challenge traditional assumptions made by medicine about both the content and role of medical work. None of these arguments have been put forward with negative intent. All are necessary to take this inquiry into the role and limits of medicine to a point where firm practical recommendations can be made. The remainder of this book seeks to extend the idea that medicine might work for health in a broad sense by suggesting how both natural and chosen limits can shape medical activity to best effect, and by suggesting how the insights generated by this process might be used to improve medical education and enhance communication between the various health professions.

However, in order that the theoretical basis for these positive suggestions can be fully understood it seems sensible to lay them out in a logical step-by-step fashion. In this way they might also be criticised more easily (although it is to be hoped that any criticism will not be based only on this precis, or only on the above summary of a theory of health which is outlined in far more detail elsewhere [56, 57]).

The 'steps so far'

These steps are not all listed in the order in which they have been presented in the book up until now. They are listed so as to make the most sense in a summarised form.

ONE
Medical interventions are always made in the context of a range of different types of uncertainty. The fullest understanding (and so the best implementation) of a medical intervention must always take account of non-clinical as well as clinical uncertainties.

TWO
The belief that it is possible to fight against disease in a *pure, reductionist fashion*, in a way which takes no account of any factor other than the disease entity or process, is clearly false. Non-clinical factors must have a part to play in the health care of human beings since it is only the very unfortunate who have no imagination or emotion, and who are unable to make judgements for themselves.

THREE
The decision to describe *any* human condition as 'normal' or 'abnormal' is always based in part on subjective judgement.

FOUR
Such subjective judging takes place whenever a decision is made to describe a person as 'diseased' or 'suffering from disease'.

Just as normality cannot be 'discovered' in a way that is entirely independent of human perception about what is to qualify as normal, so it is that the conditions that are said to be 'diseases' are not somehow objectively fixed as diseases. There is no dispute that a great deal of physiological and psychological 'dysfunctions' occur in human beings. And there is no disagreement that it is sensible to describe as 'disease' cancer in an 11-year-old boy which requires amputation of a leg. But the claim that the unwanted conditions are diseases, whether or not they are defined as such, cannot be sustained. It is simply wrong. To describe a leg as in a 'diseased condition' is an equally subjective description as to say it is in an 'unfortunate condition'.

The history of disease shows that many conditions which have been thought of as diseases are no longer so classified. What counts as a disease depends in large part on whether or not that particular *aspect of a person's life is regarded as a problem.*

FIVE
If the above steps are accepted then it becomes possible also to accept that medicine has committed an enormous theoretical mistake; a mistake which continues to have major implications for the welfare of patients. Medicine has committed a *category mistake* by *imagining* a necessary connection between health and disease. This mistake is *to regard 'health' and 'disease' as intimately linked, as if on a continuum, so that the more disease a person has the further away from perfect health he is. For those who make the category mistake 'disease' and 'health' are always related, one always depends upon the relative strength or weakness of the other.* This traditional association has been reinforced in so many ways over many years that it seems scarcely conceivable to challenge it. Yet it can be challenged, and it can be shown to be fallacious.

SIX
The steps so far result in the following scenario. Since medicine does not take place in the artificial conditions of a laboratory it has to deal with both clinical and non-clinical uncertainties. Naturally, since doctors are trained in specialist clinical techniques *their* work is against disease. However:

(1)   doctors cannot work only against disease (people have diseases);
(2)   disease does not have a higher objective status as a problem *above* other problems of life which people encounter.

But, because of tradition and generally too narrow training it is difficult for some doctors to appreciate this. These doctors continue to commit *the category mistake.*

Given the prevalence of the category mistake in medicine, it is presently the case that although doctors are not actually compelled to treat diseases there is a powerful tendency for many to believe that diseases should be tackled at almost any cost, that diseases are somehow *extraordinary problems,* problems of such a status that only when they have been eliminated do other problems become worthy of attention. The dictum '. . . there's nothing more important than your health . . .' has a powerful hold over many of us, in spite of the fact that it means many different things to different people. If it is accepted by a doctor under the spell of the category mistake it is not hard to imagine how she might emphasise disease prevention—perhaps pushing screening programmes to the point of obsession?

But this view that diseases are exceptional problems cannot be demonstrated—it is a mythical belief. Doctors have options about whether or not to intervene, and must also operate within limits which are set by non-clinical factors. Simply because a person is said to have a disease doctors are not necessarily compelled or duty-bound to treat the disease in set ways, or even at all.

Full sense can be made of the medical endeavour only when it is regarded as a *general problem-solving discipline*—a discipline which has a core body of knowledge for dealing with certain sorts of problems, but which must of necessity deal with other problems (just as is the case with any other profession). Just because medical techniques are essentially directed at disease detection, cure and prevention, this does not place disease in a class of its own as an extraordinary problem. Medicine is not an exception in this. The police force deals essentially with the maintenance of law and order and the detection of criminals, but the fact that the police exist to deal with certain categories of human problem does not make those problems so special that they must always—as a rule—take precedence over other problems. For example, the arrest of a suspected drunk driver might be abandoned in mid-course if the police officer hears that a person is in desperate need of transport to the local hospital.

All professions must deal with *perceived problems*. That is, those states perceived to be problems by the individual who suffers them, or those states perceived by others in society to be problems. This is a central insight. It is an insight which makes it possible for those who have committed the category mistake to deepen their understanding of the rationale of medical work. Once the idea is accepted that it cannot be disease *per se* that is the target for medical intervention, but must be *perceived problems*, then it becomes possible to begin to think of medicine as work for health.

The question of which and whose perceptions of problems should count as authoritative always requires careful consideration. However, to suggest a move for medicine away from a focus on disease towards a focus on *perceived problems* is an important step towards the liberation of medicine. For instance, it might suggest to Dr Clarke that the option of treating Shirley against her wishes is simply not on because she does not consider that she has a problem, even though he does.

Clearly firmer guidelines are needed to assist such difficult decisions. In order to arrive at a clearer understanding of how to order priorities in medical care conceived of as work for health, and how to set firm limits on medical activity, it is necessary to have a more extensive appreciation of the nature of health. Consequently:

SEVEN

There are several theories of health which are in competition. They contain such conflicts and incompatibilities of meaning that the theories cannot be combined into a single grand theory of health without contradiction.

EIGHT

Some of these theories of health explain health in a way that goes further than the prevention or elimination of disease and illness. However, all but one theory of health make some direct and necessary reference to disease and illness.

NINE
Although the existing theories are not fully compatible they each possess a common factor. Each theory describes work for health as work addressed essentially at the removal of obstacles to human potential (or rather conditions of life which are perceived to be obstacles). Each theory differs in its interpretation of the most valuable and most appropriate human potentials to work for in the name of health, but all recognise that the enabling of potential is the essence of health work.

TEN
Once it is accepted that there is *no logical or necessary permanent connection between work for health as enabling potentials to happen, and work against the liability of disease,* then a broader theory of health becomes a realistic option. Medical activity inspired by such a rationale must, in turn, become a broader (but by no means an unlimited) enterprise.

   This broader theory of health, a theory which sees health as the *foundations for achievement,* argues that health should not be viewed solely as the physical and mental conditions of an individual, but instead should be thought of as directly related to the conditions of life which both enable and restrict what that person can *do.* This theory can incorporate disease as a major factor in determining these life conditions, in determining what a person can do. For instance, if a person develops a cancer then her life conditions will, by and large, have changed for the worse. In order for her to regain the freedom of movement and choice she had previously her tumour must be cured. However, it is not essential to the theory of health as *foundations for achievement* that any reference to disease is made at all. For example, if a young person has in his life so far been living in a family where his mother and father frequently row, where there is little money, and where there seems to be no safe place, then, even though the young person is not diseased it still makes sense—according to several theories of health, not only the theory of health as *foundations,* to say that he is less healthy than he might be. The young man has many obstacles standing in the way of the achievement of potentials latent within him. If he had gastroenteritis, few will have difficulty recognising this as an obstacle which work for health might seek to remove. It is harder, given the current association of health with clinical goals, to see how work to provide him with a feeling of *home* can count equally as health work. But there is no reason, other than habit and bias, why it should not so count.

ELEVEN
Once the distinction between *disease and non-disease* is accepted as being both artificial and inadequate to provide a meaningful limit to medical work, the need to find some other way of demarcating health work from non-health work is obviously pressing. If doctors who wish genuinely to work for health can no longer draw the line around where their work starts and finishes, in accordance with whether or not disease is present (although very few doctors in practice ever actually do this anyway), where can they draw the line? Clearly a line must be drawn, or else doctors will be theoretically empowered—and may feel obliged—to help with every situation that a human being perceives to be a problem, which would be ludicrous.

TWELVE

As a first step, it might be said that if a doctor wishes to work for health in a way that does not depend upon either an intuitive feel for what is the right intervention to make, or upon an arbitrary distinction between disease and non-disease, then she will need to work instead with this basic rationale:

(1)   The doctor must wish in general to enable the development of potentials which will enhance the life of the subject or subjects with whom he is working.
(2)   The doctor must work to identify obstacles in the way of the development of these potentials, and choose to help with those he is best equipped to assist with. (Often this will mean that the doctor will work to fight disease and illness, although he need not confine himself to these obstacles if he feels that he might be useful.)
(3)   The doctor must avoid *dwarfing* where at all possible, and if he must dwarf, then he must do so only to avoid worse dwarfing. So, if he prescribes a drug with undesirable effects, he must do so only if not to do so will produce more undesirable effects.

Thus, three clear limits on a doctor's intervention are provisionally established. Firstly, he must identify obstacles to desirable human development. Naturally obstacles must be perceived to be obstacles, so generally speaking, even if he perceives an obstacle, he must not intervene if the subject does not perceive that his situation is problematic. Secondly, the doctor must establish that he can offer assistance. If he cannot, then this too must be a limit on his intervention. Thirdly, he must make every effort to avoid doing anything which might create fresh obstacles to desirable development.

The full answer to the question 'What should limit the doctor's activity?' rests in human autonomy rather than human disease. If health can be best understood in terms of the degree of freedom of action that a person has, then it makes far more sense to tie work for health to the notion of autonomy rather than to the notion of disease. However, autonomy is not a simple idea. In fact, there is much disagreement and confusion, amongst both philosophers and medics, about what autonomy actually is. The analysis of autonomy must be left to the second part of this book.

Part II

Limits to Medicine

Chapter Four

Models of Medicine

Now that it has been established that medicine is in one important sense a very imprecise discipline, now that traditional borders and demarcations have been demolished, it is necessary to rebuild. If medicine is not to be left in a state of theoretical anarchy—working only with the broadest theory of health—new theoretical limitations of role must be suggested. These must be coupled with the old practical limits on medical activity, which naturally still exist.

Prior to the description of a framework within which doctors might work for health whilst recognising clear limits on their practice, it is important to set the scene by briefly outlining some standard models of medicine. Each of these models has a place in medicine, but none appears to have a fully expressed philosophical rationale. As a consequence, each model becomes difficult to justify in any complete way.

It is interesting that nurses and health educators at times seem almost obsessed with 'models of nursing' or 'models of health education', whilst doctors do not seem to give a second thought to possible models of medicine. It may be that medicine is felt to be too complicated or too varied to be modelled without blatant vandalism, it may be that doctors pride themselves on action (if you can't make a diagnosis, make a decision!) above reflection about whether or not the theory on which a particular action is based is sound, or it may be that medicine is such a self-confident profession that it feels no need to explain itself by the invention of 'models of medicine'. Whatever the cause, once the analysis of medicine enters maturity—once it becomes constructive rather than aggressive—then thought through models will be required.

The classic modelling of medicine is known as 'the medical model' or 'the biomedical model'. But does such a model actually exist?

The Medical Model

The notion that medicine might have not one but several models is an unusual claim outside medical circles. Over the past two decades most critics have thought of medicine as an homogeneous discipline which can be represented fairly accurately by a single model, ubiquitously entitled 'the medical model', or the 'biomedical model' [58].

When an attempt is made to characterise 'the medical model' by use of a single coherent description, the model looks hugely naive to those who are involved in medical practice. Below is a standard version of 'the medical model', limited to the most typically mentioned features. The model is presented, as it usually is, to include both implicit and explicit criticism of medicine. Indeed, the phrase 'the medical model' is commonly used euphemistically for more choice expressions, such as 'elitist', 'paternalist', 'arrogant', 'technology-obsessed', or 'overpaid profession'!

'Medicine is now so dominated by science and technology that it is driven more by the thirst for new knowledge, and the desire to discover ever more sophisticated techniques, than it is by the aim to care for the "whole person". The emphasis on science leads inexorably to a preoccupation with measurement, to a tunnel vision which regards only the quantifiable aspects of human beings as significant. And this attitude, in turn, "dehumanises" doctors so that they do not see themselves as "helping people", but believe instead that their task is to return bodies to normal function, rather in the way that a plumber seeks to rejuvenate a central heating system by replacing the water pump. Without a focus on "the whole person" doctors assume paternalist attitudes whereby they think they know what is "in the patient's best interest" better than the patient.

Doctors consume large amounts of a nation's financial resources, often in the pursuit of esoteric and often quite useless research. This research is rarely "pure inquiry". The form it takes is shaped by various interests, but often primarily by the priorities of the powerful pharmaceutical industry. Thus, funding is far more likely for a drug which would be widely purchased than for one which would benefit only a small group of people, and so would not justify the investment necessary for its development. In addition, medicine's pursuit of better clinical knowledge must be set in a social context where the primary causes of most disease and illness are not "accidental dysfunction", but an avoidable result of living in societies which perpetuate gross inequalities of wealth and power.'

There is truth within these criticisms, some of which has spilt over into the argument of this book, but there is also considerable misrepresentation.

What is wrong with the naive version of the medical model? The following points should be thought of as initial criticism, not of the content of the above account but of the assumption that such a model can possibly be an adequate description of reality:

(1) Doctors practise medicine within separate specialisms. Although the 50-year-old psychiatrist, who is a strong advocate of psychotherapy, may have learnt his medicine at the same medical school at the same time as the 50-year-old Professor of Pharmacology and Therapeutics, to say that they both espouse precisely the same 'medical model' must be demonstrably wrong. The two doctors practise their medicine in different ways, and apparently in accord with quite different tenets. One will use drugs only as a last resort, the other sees drug therapy as central to the medical endeavour.

(2) There are differences in the interpretation of the role of medicine made by doctors from different eras. Although it is possible that their views will be quite harmonious it is likely that 25-year-old and 55-year-old doctors will have different outlooks in some respects, and that over at least some questions concerning appropriate medical practice they will disagree. For example, the older doctor is more likely than the younger to adopt a paternalist style [59]. In part these differences will be the result of their developing in different historical periods—attitudes towards doctors are far less reverential now than they once were [60]. In part the differences over time will be the result of changes in technology (the younger doctor needs to learn more technical skills), and in part as a result of developments in medical education.

(3) An argument advanced by some social scientists is that medical schools tend not only to 'professionalise' but also to 'socialise' medical students. This is a fairly powerful argument. In essence it asserts that medical schools actually do much more than train students to perform to the accepted standards of their professional group. In a variety of ways medical schools mould, encourage, and pressurise young people into *whole lives*—not just working lives. It is argued that in order for a person to become a doctor—in order for him to be an accepted member of a profession—he must conform to the basic 'role model' of a doctor. By and large he will be middle-class, and generally be an adherent of THE medical model. Usually without knowing it he will be an 'agent of social control', and himself be a pawn in the grand design perpetuating social order [61].

But this belief rests on too much abstraction from reality. Although, broadly speaking, it may be true that non-conformist students tend to be weeded out, none the less it is an inadequate assumption that the young people are not exposed to other important influences in life, and that these must also have a bearing on the role they will assume, the model they will most identify with, and the limits of practice they will accept.

The assumption that there is such a thing as THE medical model is too crude. What are the standard alternatives? [62]

Each of the models described below are also abstractions. It is not suggested that doctors who conform perfectly to these models actually exist. On viewing the models most doctors will recognise that they and their colleagues are amalgams of two or more. But whatever the 'mix' from which a particular doctor believes he is constructed it is likely that he will lean more towards one model than any other. And there will be those who recognise a model as at least a reasonable approximation to the beliefs and practices of someone known to them. However, it is suggested that none of these models has the credibility of the theory that medical work should be thought of in terms of work for health.

Alternative Models?

In this section four possible alternative models of medical practitioner are described. The four models are entitled the *Purist*, the *Mechanic*, the *Carer*, and the *Guardian*.

A realistic assessment of the practical drives of any of the models must include impulses to action such as personal ambition and satisfaction, and financial gain for the scientist and his department. The extent to which these practical drives influence the work of the doctor will vary with each doctor and each context.

The Purist

The typical *Purist* is a clinical researcher (and so not necessarily a doctor of medicine). The *Purist* has particular sympathy with the first part of THE medical model. He or she will, through the application of scientific principles and techniques, attempt to work to discover more precise knowledge of the functioning of the human body, and of its reaction to various stimuli. The *Pure* medic attempts to contribute to the general task of increasing pharmacological knowledge by researching into the properties, applications and efficacy of drugs. The *Purist* has only a secondary concern with the welfare of patients as people—interventions on patients are made with the intention of *contributing to medical knowledge* as the primary professional object.

The central theoretical drive of the *Pure* model might be said to be this: *that above all else medicine must be scrupulously scientific.* Protocols must be rigorous, samples must be comprehensive, hypotheses must be precise, and trials must always be controlled (i.e. tests must be carried out on subjects, but their reactions must be assessed not only in terms of changes in these subjects, but in terms of the continuing state of carefully matched controls who are not the subjects of the test procedure).

For the strict adherent to the *Pure* model the extent to which medicine can be said to be *real* medicine must be judged according to the extent to which it conforms to accepted scientific standards. Any medical activity which cannot be identified with these ideals (for instance where a doctor offers health promotion advice in a primary care setting) is not at the core of medicine, but only a secondary task.

Useful knowledge can be generated by the *Purist*. For instance, research in pharmacology can produce drugs which not only assist in 'disease' cure, but produce associated benefit for other models. To give just one example, the clinical researcher Black [63] produced a drug (cimetidine) which blocks acid secretion. This discovery has reduced problems caused by stomach ulcers, and in turn has taken some pressure of work from surgeons and general practitioners.

However, absolute *Purity* in medicine is a false hope. The *Pure* model can only ever be hypothetical because clinical research is never, ultimately, pure. Consider the following points:

(1) Experiments carried out in laboratory conditions produce results which are not necessarily replicated when methods or treatments are applied to people in real life [64]. This is especially true of experiments involving animals [65].

(2) Within a range of possibility there can be very different reactions to the same surgical or drug interventions [66].

(3) It is possible to overemphasise the importance of pure research. On occasions this overemphasis is a result of *the category mistake*. Some *Purists* can seem to be driven by a desire to discover knowledge for the sake of knowing, without asking whether it is truly important to know [67]. Indeed, there are some things that we may not wish to know. For example, we may decide that it is wrong to know the degree of pain that a child can bear before death is inevitable, even though such knowledge might, conceivably, be useful. In this way ethical considerations can rightly corrupt the *Pure* model by indicating that some research is morally unacceptable.

Sometimes research is repeated, even though the chances are that earlier research evidence is probably true. One unfortunate example of this occurred in Papua New Guinea, where a controlled trial was carried out giving iodine supplement to some tribes people in order to see if this lowered the incidence of cretinism. It did—dramatically—but earlier (known) research indicated that this would be the case. On one interpretation it could be said that some of the offspring of the control group (those who suffered cretinism) were sacrificed to the interests of pure research [68].

(4) Much 'knowledge' generated by *Pure* research is ephemeral—soon superseded or shown to be mistaken, or misguided [69].

Some limits of the model The strict *Purist* is both enabled and limited by the rigour of science. Thus, although he operates with very clear guidelines and tight methodology which allow him a high degree of precision, he will usually be able to concentrate on only a very small facet of clinical work. In other words, his science allows him to become an accurate specialist only in the smallest area. His area of competence may be only (metaphorically speaking) the underside of the left big toe. The *Purist* will be competitive with other workers with exact knowledge of the toe, and will find it difficult to work in teams.

But more than this, it is not clear why—apart from the obvious practical and personal incentives to be successful—the *Purist* does what he does. Apart from adherence to an heroic notion of scientific idealism (an idea which has been thoroughly discredited by work in the philosophy of science [70]) it is not clear what the values and underpinning theory of the *Purist* are.

The Mechanic

Although 'THE medical model' is a caricature, and cannot be taken properly to represent the enormous complexity and diversity of the medical endeavour, elements of it retain a certain truth. Just as doctors can be found who fit the description (more or less) of the *Pure* clinician, so others can be found who might be described as fitting the *Mechanic* model.

The *Mechanic* is a type of doctor who thinks purely in physical terms. Judged by their explanation of illness some general practitioners are *Mechanics*, but the model is more appropriate to surgeons and physicians (hospital doctors). This is not necessarily a critical comment. In part it is precisely the nature of the surgeon's work that he is a mechanic, working as he does with mechanical parts and mechanical theories. And, as with every other stereotypical role offered in this section, to adhere to this model of medicine is to make a legitimate choice of medical role—even though this choice of model does not permit the doctor to express clearly the theoretical inspiration for the selection (and so does not enable the visualisation of clear limits to medical intervention).

The *Mechanic* is concerned to combat deviations from the accepted norm for physical systems. He is generally a very practical person who seeks to apply his skills to the removal of obstacles to physical development, for example as a surgeon removes a tumour. The *Mechanic* is usually a doctor who thinks in terms of clear disease entities. He is less at home with abstract notions of illness—or when attempting to work in areas where emotion and feeling come into play.

Some limits of the model The *Mechanic* may find himself particularly limited by lack of resources. For instance, he may find that he has no organ available to transplant, no bed for a patient, or a limit on the budget he has available. Developments in technology tend to expand the extent of the possible for the *Mechanic* while limited funding contracts it.

Like all the models the *Mechanic* is generally limited by considerations of ethics [71]. However, it is most likely that he will see himself specifically rather than generally constrained. Like the *Purist*, who will often feel that he is limited only by a particular branch of ethics—namely *research ethics*—the *Mechanic* can believe that he is constrained only by the need to obtain informed consent for any procedure he wishes to carry out. But this is far from the truth. It is argued in detail, in several parts of this book, that all doctors who seek to help people achieve health should seek to enable as many potentials as possible. Thus, although it may be regarded as a minimum ethical requirement, it will rarely be enough for the surgeon brusquely to obtain a signature on a consent form. If the opportunity existed to enable a patient to understand more, and to feel more secure (if indeed she has reason to), then the doctor ought to have made the most of it.

The Carer

Practitioners of this model of medicine, in contrast to the *Purist* and the *Mechanic*, regard the essential role of medicine as being 'to offer human care—to offer medical care only if it is possible to care for a person as a whole'. This quotation is illustrative of the genre.

> '(Tom) is one of the forgotten ones, marginalised in the inner city. Being male makes it worse: he has no small child to make him the subject of case conferences and continuing support. Who would really care if he took an overdose tomorrow?
>
> I would care. I'm fond of Tom. I want him to get his O-Level. I want him to be content. I suffer to see him unhappy. This morning I gave him some thioridazine (a strong but non-addictive tranquilliser) to calm him down and help him sleep. I'm sure we can sort out his electricity, and some petty cash from the practice will enable him to eat for the next few days. More and more I am coming to see that as my role. I am the last resort. When other agencies wash their hands I have to remain the befriender.' [72].

Taken from a magazine article, this is a clear statement of what it means to be a *Caring* medic.

The *Carer* will have a strong desire, even a need, to empathise with his patients, and will often have some ability to do so. The *Carer* will usually be able to obtain a reasonable insight into the perceptions, anxieties and hopes of the person he wishes to help.

The *Carer* who wishes to empathise, but who is not gifted with insight into other people, is a disastrous doctor. The *Carer* will often seek to help in areas which are not clinical and for which he has no special training. It is possible that the *Carer* will geniunely see himself both as a professional and as a voluntary worker! The *Carer* will have an urge to give. He will, at times, actually 'suffer with' his patients, and will hope not only to be appreciated but actually to be liked.

Doctors who fit the *Carer* model of medicine, whilst offering a clinical service (offering appropriate treatment and therapy) also tend to emphasise the essentially human aspects of their care of patients. The *Carer* will tend to ask 'But how do *you* feel?', 'Would you like to talk about it?', and will probably feel able to touch patients, or even to cry with them. The *Carer* has a view of medicine centred on 'the person' rather than science. He will seek to pay attention to every aspect of a person's life, not just those aspects found in standard medical textbooks. Consequently, in contrast to the more clinical *Purist* or *Mechanic*, the *Carer* can be of benefit in a wide range of ways—from help with housing, a marriage, or an emotional crisis, to prescribing an effective anti-inflammatory agent for lumbago.

The *Carer* might have any of the set of clinical skills, but by dint of personality will have been more inclined as a student to enter the 'softer' disciplines of medicine. So, in addition to basic clinical know-how, the *Carer* will be adept at communication, at listening, perhaps at counselling, and—importantly—will have become a specialist in advocacy. In other words the *Carer* will be inclined to speak up for the weak, the vulnerable, the powerless—when they are unable to do so for themselves. Advocacy is currently an activity which is especially favoured by some members of the nursing profession who feel that many patients need advocates [73]. Some nurses feel that patients need advocates to speak for them against their doctors, whilst the *Carer* believes that doctors should also be advocates. Fortunately this does not necessarily imply confrontation between advocates since the *Caring* doctor tends to share many of the attributes traditionally associated with the nursing profession. In addition, the role of the advocate doctor is less to advocate for the patient within hospital and more to advocate for the patient within society. Where external circumstances are seen to be unfairly stacked against a person it is here that the *Carer* believes he has a role, regardless of whether or not the assistance is within the clinical realm, and regardless of whether the *Carer* has been trained in the skill.

The person-centred model has disadvantages. For example, the *Carer* may be drawn too much into collusion with the plans of patients rather than seek to offer the most creative care. It may be that by agreeing to sign a person off sick with a 'viral illness', or by agreeing to continue the existing dose of Valium because of the 'tension in our house', the best policy is not implemented. Sometimes it can be better to identify other potentials with the patient, and then try to make these into a reality.

All *Carers* have been reared in the environment of *Purists* and *Mechanics*. They have been raised in a culture where to succeed a doctor or medical student must be disease-centred rather than person-centred, reductionist rather than holist. And this causes unease in the *Carer* who takes the view that people and diseases are significantly different, and who might even claim the slogan 'there are no diseases, only people with problems!'.

Some limits of the model Although practicalities such as resources, law and language must limit the activities of the *Carer*, perhaps the most significant limits are those of competence and ethics. It may be that the good intentions of the *Carer* turn out to be counterproductive if these limits are not recognised. It may be that the Carer attempts to intervene when the work might be better left to other caring agencies, although she will be inclined towards an approach which shares uncertainties not only with patients but with other caring agencies. And, in addition, the consequences of her caring so much might be unintended dependency (Will Tom come to rely on her too heavily? Will he see her as a soft touch?), a waste of her expensively produced clinical skills, and a 'patching up' of a social system which some *Carers* regard as one of the causes of the problem in the first place.

The Guardian

The *Guardian* is quite closely related to the *Carer*, but where the *Carer* is primarily concerned to take individual people under his wing the *Guardian* seeks to protect society. The (self-appointed) role of the *Guardian* is to work in the public interest—to protect the 'public health'. *Guardians* tend to see themselves as special, as having a radically different role to other professionals. Whereas a lawyer, or an architect, may have broad concerns (say with justice or with the aesthetics of the environment) he will, at bottom, be promoting the particular interests of his client. Thus, he will inevitably represent special interests. Indeed he will take on some of the values of the person for whom he is working. But the *Guardian* sees himself to be a creature of a different kind. Typically his view is this.

> Since the *Guardian* is a medic he is essentially a scientist with humanitarian interests. Since he is a scientist then his task is not to represent the views of particular people but first to observe and record the prevailing state of affairs, and then second to do something to improve this state of affairs in the interest of vulnerable people.

According to the *Guardian* this is not a contradictory argument because of a very special reason—at least a special reason in the eyes of the *Guardian*. The *Guardian* does not see himself as promoting the special interest of individuals or even groups of individuals. Unlike other professionals the *Guardian* is working for health, and health is not something that is a value, or desired, or a good thing only for some people and not others. On the contrary, health is universally desired, and so it is possible for the guardian to seek to promote health without any danger of being embroiled in special pleading.

Essentially the medic as *Guardian* believes she is unique among professionals, because she is neutral. It is most likely that the *Guardian* will be an expert in community or public health, with a background in epidemiology. She will regard herself as an applied scientist with the special task to serve. In addition to the belief in her neutrality the *Guardian* reveres two key measures. These measures are morbidity and mortality—the incidence of sickness and the incidence of death. They are part and parcel of the view that medicine, at least in the form practised by the *Guardian*, is a neutral endeavour: surely no-one wants to be sick and no-one wants to die.

The main advantage of the approach of the *Guardian* is that clear pictures can be established over populations of the pattern in which diseases and illnesses are manifested. In theory this should allow the most effective targeting of both preventive and curative measures. But in practice it is far from simple. Studies into the 'public health' have shown that in different parts of the country diseases and deaths occur at different rates, and that the same applies for different social classes [74]. These findings transmit the supposedly neutral *Guardian* into the arena of political controversy. Not only are the findings disputed, but so are conclusions about the causation of these inequalities, and even the methods of both research and analysis [75].

Some limits of the model   It is a fallacy to believe that it is possible to work for health as a neutral. People disagree about what social priorities should be brought into being in the interest of the health of populations. The basic difficulty lies in the realm of ethics since 'the public interest' is a many faceted idea. Values conflict so that it is hardly ever, if at all, possible to work for public health without causing one party or another to be aggrieved. Consider this brief example.

In the winter of 1988/89 there was a widely publicised 'egg scare'. A junior health minister claimed that most egg production was infected with salmonella, a bacteria which can cause sickness and even death. Naturally people were alarmed and many stopped eating eggs, which in turn alarmed the egg producers. It was argued by some that the state of chicken and egg production was scandalous and showed how little regard farmers and the government have for the 'public health' (to say nothing of the health of the chickens). Consequently it was asserted that public health inspectors and veterinary surgeons should test chickens for the presence of salmonella, and if infection was found should destroy the flock.

But here is one example of a clash of interest. Scientific research shows what the facts are, but it is a mistake (and is the mistake of the *Guardian* who believes that he is a neutral) to believe that just because all the scientific evidence leads to one conclusion about the current state of affairs, that all points of view will lead with the same degree of certainty to one conclusion about what is to be done. The *Guardian* actually has to make a choice. He has to choose between the risk of food poisoning in vulnerable groups such as the very young and the very old, and the risk of depression and other illness in farmers, their workers, and their families.

The *Guardian* doesn't just report.

He decides what to research in the first place (i.e. he makes a positive choice).
He decides what to do with the information when he has gathered it.
He makes judgements about what is in the public interest based not on scientific criteria, but on the basis of certain values that he and his colleagues hold.

Summary

This section on models of medicine, although partly light-hearted, was meant to drive home a serious point, and to demonstrate that in order for this inquiry to offer practical help to doctors more precision is necessary. None of these 'models' is at all adequate to represent medical activity comprehensively and in a way which might enable a deeper understanding of its rationale.

Contrary to the mythology of social science there is not only a single medical or biomedical model. Medicine is such a diverse enterprise—and the members of the profession have such varied inspirations—that it cannot adequately be fitted into theoretical boxes at all. There are trends, and there are exceptions to every trend.

However, just because medicine cannot be characterised adequately this does not mean that the key questions '*What role ought a doctor adopt?*', '*What things must limit a doctor's activity?*' and '*What's medicine for?*' are empty questions which no-one can hope to answer. On the contrary these are central difficulties for medicine as a whole, and for the individual doctor in her daily work. Should I listen to this patient telling me about her husband's jealousy? Should I encourage the teenage girl to return in two weeks to tell me if her stepfather has made more advances, or should I tell the police? Should I perform a minor operation or should I refer? Should I diagnose depression or should I keep quiet, not wishing to upset the patient?

Should I prescribe the antidepressant made by the drug company which sponsors the annual meeting?

Should I tell the patient that he has cancer? Should I tell the relatives? How can I communicate with this younger man? Should I help this single parent with the form for Housing Benefit? Should I offer this person this very expensive treatment or not?

These are real problems for doctors which cannot be solved merely by selecting one basic model or another. More is required to be helpful. At the very least it is necessary to have:

(1)   A deeper understanding of the rationale of medicine—a firm grasp of why it is that medical work is a valuable occupation, and an occupation of a radically different kind to other professions.
(2)   A means to imagine, in a graphic way, how close—in specific contexts and circumstances—the doctor is to the limits of his capacity. It is important for doctors to be able to judge, however crudely, how confident they ought to be about each intervention they are proposing to carry out. To this end the next section introduces the idea of *Rings of Uncertainty*, and develops this idea so that it becomes possible for doctors to score, albeit roughly, how near to the limits they are.

A number of limits to each model have been indicated, but the present picture is abstract, hypothetical and messy. It is time to consider a more realistic modelling of medical practice—one which works very clearly to display limits and suggests a practical way of ordering priorities.

Exercise Three

Which Hat Should I Wear?

This exercise is designed to help doctors consider which roles to adopt when there are alternatives, and there is doubt.

The potential suicide and the Accident and Emergency Consultant

This is an apparently straightforward exercise. A scenario is presented which causes a problem for a doctor, in this case, a consultant in Accident and Emergency. Once the scene has been set a range of options for care are outlined; these are roughly in accord with the four models of medicine discussed in this chapter. The basic task of the exercise is:

(1)   to decide which option will liberate the most enhancing human potential in this situation,
(2)   to decide whether or not the selected option conforms to a legitimate role for a professional clinician,
(3)   to justify answers to (1) and (2),
(4)   and if no justification can be given to begin to consider better alternatives.

continued on next page

continued

Irene's despair

It is Saturday night in the Casualty Department of a provincial city hospital. It is eight o'clock and not yet the busiest time for the Department. Christopher Evans, a middle-aged consultant in Accident and Emergency is talking to a colleague at the reception desk when Irene rushes in, obviously in great distress. She stands unsteadily and her eyes are wide and wild. She spots Christopher, who lives in the same street as her.

"I am going to kill myself, and I want as many people as I can to see me, and to know why I am killing myself."

She draws breath and goes on, "Brian has been unfaithful. He's cheated on me. Not once but often and it's gone on for years now. I can't stand it any more. He treats me like dirt. He makes me feel worthless. All he cares about is himself and his own pleasure. I put everything into our marriage. I have nothing without it. But our marriage is nothing.

I don't want to live like this any longer. I want him to pay. I want him to suffer like I've suffered. It's his fault that I am going to kill myself, and I want him to feel the guilt. I want you to tell him that he's killed me."

Now sobbing, Irene forces a handful of white pills into her mouth, opens a half-empty bottle of whiskey, and swallows the pills. Christopher is transfixed, as are the 20 or so other people in the waiting room—a doctor, two nurses, a receptionist and patients. Irene sits down purposefully on a chair in the middle of the room and puts her head in her hands. She begins to rock gently forwards and back again.

Christopher is not easily shocked, but he is surprised to see Irene in such a state. From the casual chats that he has had with her over the years he had no idea that she was suffering torment. Christopher knew Irene as a quiet housewife of a professional man, in her late forties, with two teenage boys. She was always pleasant.

Now Christopher has a major decision to make. What, if anything, should he do to help Irene? Which model of practice is most appropriate? These seem to be the options:

The doctor as Purist

Christopher Evans the *Purist* might decide that a suicide attempt is not the concern of medical doctors. It might be possible to save Irene's life, assuming that she has taken an overdose of paracetamol, since there is an effective antidote. But since she does not wish to take it, she should be seen by a priest, not by a doctor whose time could be better spent working with people who wish to live.

Alternatively, the *Purist* might decide to observe Irene as she dies, recording her physical and mental condition as she progresses towards unconsciousness. This might be useful scientific data, although of a rather qualitative kind.

Issues

- Although the *Purist* might appear callous, he is quite clear about his role as a doctor. He is clear that his responsibility lies with patients who need him, and with the future, rather than with someone who has evidently done with living—is such clarity justifiable?

continued on next page

continued

• Is the *Purist* running any risks, in any sense of the word (e.g. a risk to his conscience, a risk of not delivering a proper level of care, a risk to his credibility with other staff)?

The doctor as Mechanic

Christopher Evans the *Mechanic* might take a different line. Here is just one option that might be considered. The *raison d'être* of the *Mechanic* is to prevent or cure disease and illness. The *Mechanic* judges his success and failure in terms of things that can be measured, and his standard measures are morbidity and mortality. Christopher Evans the *Mechanic* has a preventable mortality on his hands. Thus he sees his role quite clearly. He cannot sit back and allow a patient (*is* she his patient?) to die before his eyes. Consequently, he force-feeds her the antidote and places her under nursing supervision until she can be properly assessed by a psychiatrist.

Issues

• Where does Christopher Evans the *Mechanic* stand legally?
• Where does he stand morally?

The doctor as Carer

Christopher Evans the *Carer* might see himself as having yet another role (the *Carer* may well see more than the single role outlined here). Like Christopher Evans the *Mechanic*, Christopher Evans the *Carer* cannot stand by and watch Irene die. But rather than force her to live the *Carer* will counsel, support, and persuade in a subtle way. Through listening and talking and befriending the *Carer* will hope to save a life. Naturally it is open to any *Carer* (or any other of the hypothetical models) to *change* role in mid-crisis. Perhaps the *Carer* will become the *Mechanic* if things become desperate.

Issues

• Is Christopher the *Carer* more vulnerable than Christopher the *Mechanic*, for instance?
• Is there a point at which a doctor should not expose himself to harm?
• Is it an appropriate professional role for a doctor to *suffer* for or with his patients?

The doctor as Guardian

Christopher Evans the *Guardian* might take a more lofty approach. His experience may have hardened him to death. Dying people are part of his life and he will not intervene in a suicide attempt if he can find no evidence of mental illness, or unless the person asks for his help. He will not take the fact that Irene has come to a Casualty Department as evidence that she wants to be saved because she has said that what she wants is publicity, not help. *Wilson* v. *Pringle* [76] notwithstanding he believes that he has no legal right to touch another person without her consent.

However, the *Guardian* is chairing a Regional Health Authority working group on public health provision. This group, the great majority of whom are medics, consider that they have a very wide brief to recommend interventions in the 'public interest'.

continued on next page

continued

Such interventions include raising the price of tobacco and alcohol, rigorous screening programmes for disease which people must 'opt out' of rather than volunteer for, compulsory vaccination for school children, and preventive adult-education programmes designed to help people cope better should they ever feel suicidal.

Issues
- If this level of intervention is acceptable for 'the public health' how is not intervening to stop one individual death not also justifiable?
- Is this Christopher Evans doing enough for Irene in the circumstances?
- Is there a role, a model, or alternative option, which ought to be advanced but has not been suggested by this exercise?

Chapter Five

The Rings of Uncertainty

Introduction

Given that doctors might wish, and in practice often do wish, to work for health in a sense which goes beyond work against disease, how might they assess their most appropriate roles? How might they decide when not to intervene, or when they should cease to intervene? This chapter suggests a beginning. It offers a way for doctors to picture their positions in a world of uncertainty. It is intended that by means of this *picturing* doctors will be better placed to judge the most desirable courses to take.

Recall the key questions of this inquiry. The investigation began with the puzzles '*What role ought a doctor adopt?*' and '*To what extent should a doctor intervene—what should limit a doctor's activity?*' At present doctors are guided primarily by precedent and subjective judgement, both in general and in particular contexts. There exists no substantial framework of thinking to help a medic arrive at a more systematic reasoned position. And because of this lack it is often difficult for others—doctors, other health carers, and patients—to challenge the reasoning process which led to an intervention. It is still the case that the vague phrase 'I exercised my clinical judgement' is sometimes used to conceal woolly or dubious reasoning. Other health professionals have no shared framework to enable either encouragement or restraint. If a nurse thinks that a doctor is not doing enough to help a patient, or a manager believes that a doctor is going too far, there is no general logical framework to facilitate discussion. Confrontation often occurs where instead there might have been constructive conversation.

This part of the book tries to change this situation for the better. By presenting a graphic, graspable model for doctors to reflect upon possible roles and interventions this chapter offers a way for doctors to increase further their understanding of the philosophical basis of their work. It also suggests a means of enhancing communication between doctors and other health workers—to the benefit of those who are cared for. The framework presented in the following pages is not meant to be dogmatic but to help enhance the deliberations of doctors. Very many decisions taken in health care contexts inevitably fall within the province of personal judgement, for which there are seemingly indefinite methodologies. It is rarely the case in health care that there is only one answer to a problem. Usually there are alternative possibilities, each of which will have merit. However, there are limits which distinguish acceptable answers from the unacceptable. The *Rings of Uncertainty* and the *Autonomy Test* (which is explained in the following chapter) are designed to reveal clear limits beyond which doctors ought not act. These devices help display the boundaries to medical practice. It is argued in this chapter that doctors should not transcend these boundaries, although they should have a high degree of liberty within them.

Limits

Not one but several limits restrict medical practice. These limits are bound always to be present, even though their breadth and specification might change. For example, limits of technical competence, limits set by legislation, and various limits of language will inevitably set boundaries for medicine.

Given that these limits obviously exist in medicine, and given the deep uncertainty about where these general limits ought to have force in specific contexts, a guiding framework should be a welcome development. If doctors can accept that uncertainty impregnates all aspects of medicine it becomes possible to employ this reality to set a guide for thinking about the best forms of care. The general title for this guide for the imagination is the *Rings of Uncertainty*. The Rings can best be explained in a series of steps.

The Rings of Uncertainty

Step One

Uncertainty is the most abiding and pervasive limit on medical activity. Uncertainty in medicine can be generally represented in the graphic fashion shown in Figure 5.1.

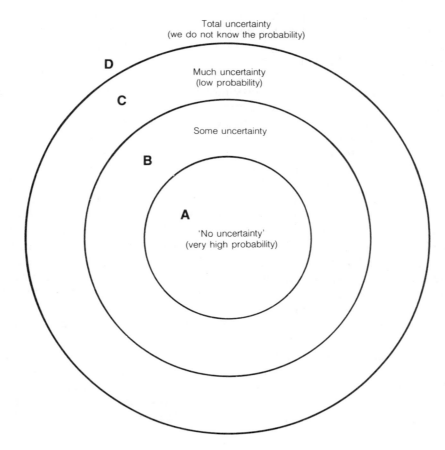

Total uncertainty
(we do not know the probability)

D

Much uncertainty
(low probability)

C

Some uncertainty

B

A

'No uncertainty'
(very high probability)

Figure 5.1

Traditionally the aim of the medical endeavour is to move from the outside to the inside, to move ever closer to certainty. However, when this abstract model is expressed in more specific terms it can be seen that this inward progress is not necessarily always the most appropriate course for medicine as work for health—for a liberating medicine—to plot.

It is not always undesirable for the doctor to move outwards. For some expressions of the Rings the best policy might be to experiment with various positions. On occasions it could be argued that the doctor—particularly if he thinks of himself as a general problem-solver who wishes to work for health—ought to try to move into the outer rings. Although this may not be the safest option—for instance, it becomes more likely that he will be exposed to criticism—there are considerable benefits which might be gained. For example, by stretching outwards the doctor might learn from other people and so extend her personal range of competence; she might discover fresh and broader options for problem-solving; new approaches and methodologies might become apparent; and—perhaps most importantly of all—by welcoming the idea of outward travel rather than constantly seeking shelter in certainty, her flexibility may increase. She may learn when to be humble, and—when appropriate—to be passive rather than active. Indeed it is only by facing outwards as well as in that the doctor can work for health in the richest sense [77].

The crude model drawn above can be adapted for any of the major limits on medical practice. In this way the Rings can be given meaning. As an initial example, consider the Rings expressed in terms of technical competence.

Step Two: the Rings expressed

Technical competence

Technical competence includes both knowledge and skill. Competence (or lack of it) might be expressed in various ways. Here in Figure 5.2 is one translation of the idea of technical competence into the form of the Rings of Uncertainty.

As is the case with all general guiding frameworks the words used to describe each Ring can mean different things dependent upon particular circumstances. For instance, the competencies in question might be competencies of technique, or recall of information. And when the Rings are expressed in terms of resources these might be human organs, money, beds, time, or skilled people—whatever might legitimately be considered to be a resource. Reality must give meaning to each Ring.

Figure 5.2 shows a simple representation of one way in which medical activity might be imagined to be limited by competence. It is better not to imagine a doctor jumping from one section of the Rings to another. Although the Rings appear to be sharply divided as they are illustrated, in reality different levels of competence shade into each other, just as a bold scarlet can fade slowly to the palest pink. The Rings are meant to transmit an image of a steady weakening of certainty—a weakening of competence in the present case—as the doctor moves towards the outer edge. It is expected that certain questions are likely to arise dependent upon the doctor's perceived position. For example, is the doctor the only person in a position to offer help? Should the doctor intervene only with the advice and assistance of others? Is the doctor's ability to help so limited that any intervention by him is inappropriate?

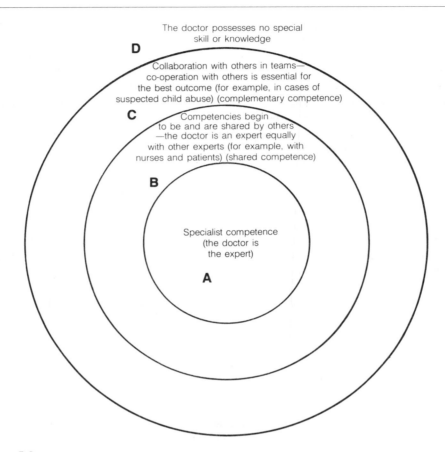

D The doctor possesses no special skill or knowledge

C Collaboration with others in teams—co-operation with others is essential for the best outcome (for example, in cases of suspected child abuse) (complementary competence)

B Competencies begin to be and are shared by others—the doctor is an expert equally with other experts (for example, with nurses and patients) (shared competence)

A Specialist competence (the doctor is the expert)

Figure 5.2

A doctor within the Rings: a practical example in terms of technical competence

Imagine how Dr Clarke, the doctor who had a patient he suspected to be anorexic, might have made use of the Rings, picturing himself both actually and potentially within them. As Dr Clarke thought and began to confront uncertainty he had a perplexing array of practical choices. By using the Rings he could have placed these choices in a general graphic context. The Rings make it possible for a doctor to reason in a more concrete way. It becomes possible to say 'If I do *that*, then I shall be standing in this position within the Rings of Uncertainty'. In one sense this is to do no more than to say 'if I do this, then X will happen', but the option to refer to an image can create deeper thinking and insight than merely asking 'What if . . . ?' questions unaided. The doctor must introspect and test proposals against fact in either case. At the very least *picturing* can do no harm.

Dr Clarke began at one position within the Rings. He had the option to move if he chose, but he was not entirely free to place himself wherever he wished. As Shirley's case developed, external events—circumstances beyond Dr Clarke's control—had the effect of moving him within the Rings. If Shirley had attempted suicide, for instance, this would have affected his position within the Rings expressed in terms of competence. Could the doctor have coped with this situation? However, it remains true to say that, to a greater or lesser extent dependent upon circumstances, the position in which a doctor *chooses* to place himself will influence the outcome of his intervention for the patient. The doctor is faced with certain basic questions. How far should I extend my influence? Which position am I *able* to occupy? Which part of the circles should I decide to occupy? Always there must be an interplay between uncertainties of fact (What will happen if X is done?) and uncertainties of perception (Am I competent enough to do X?).

When Shirley and her mother first consulted, Dr Clarke felt secure within the central area of the Rings expressed in terms of competence. He was behind his desk, in his surgery, with his books and technological assistance. He felt equipped to deal with most of the cases who might walk in—and those he did not feel able to deal with he could always refer on to specialists (so bypassing the Rings, leaping directly into the outer area surrounding the rings).

But Dr Clarke soon discovered that Shirley presented a problem requiring thorough deliberation if the most beneficial outcome were to be achieved. He recognised quickly that he needed at least initial help with Shirley, at which point he moved into the second circle—where competencies are shared by others. The advice he then received forced him to consider in turn:

(1) placing himself back within *the centre* **(A)**. The senior partner thought that Dr Clarke could, and should, take full responsibility for the situation himself.
(2) moving to the *outer surrounding area* **(D)**, by referring Shirley to the psychiatrist—an option he considered in anger.
(3) moving to *the perimeter ring* **(C)**, by working in collaboration with others, including Shirley as a full member of the team—as Dr Green suggested.

In fact Dr Clarke finally decided to settle for Dr Green's advice. He recognised that he was quite unable to operate alone since he would have been outside the Rings. Any attempt to do so would have ended in disaster—a clear limit on the medical assistance that he was able to offer. His difficulty—expressed metaphorically—was to find the correct area of the Rings to operate within for that patient in that context. This is always a fundamental issue whenever a doctor seeks to work for the health of a patient.

Other expressions

The same Rings of Uncertainty—stretching from a core where confidence can be at a peak to a surrounding area where there is no ground for any professional intervention—can be translated into several major categories. The possible designations of category are almost endless. Doctors will be free to suggest their own labels if they find the general idea of the Rings of Uncertainty helpful. However, although by no means an exclusive list, the following additional categories are suggested in addition to that of technical competence.

Resources

Broader picturing: *resources plus technical competence*
Naturally any analysis undertaken by a doctor within the real-life environment of uncertainty is far more complex than the simple picture of Dr Clarke moving only within the Rings expressed in terms of technical competence.

The following brief example (Figure 5.3) shows how complexity can begin to deepen. Imagine Dr Smith, a consultant surgeon standing within the *Rings of Uncertainty* expressed in terms of resources. In order for him to work to greatest effect, to direct his time and energy along the most profitable channels, it is necessary for him to understand his position correctly within the Rings expressed in this way. Clearly, where he is able to stand will vary dependent upon the extent of the resources available, and might also change according to the interpretation he gives to the word 'resource'.

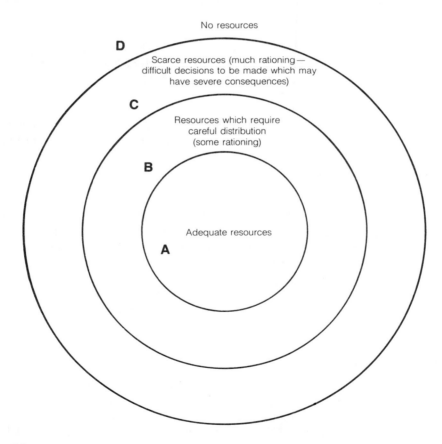

Figure 5.3

In order to arrive at the best practical approach to his problem it will usually be necessary for Dr Smith to see himself standing simultaneously within other expressions of the *Rings of Uncertainty*: as if two or more Rings were superimposed one on another. For instance, if the surgeon wishes to perform a heart transplant then it is certain that there will be issues of resource. But inevitably there will be other variables to consider, of which technical competence will be one.

As far as resources are concerned, if there is no suitable donor organ available, then Dr Smith will be stranded in *the area surrounding the Rings* **(D)**. If a compatible heart does become available, then Dr Smith will either be operating within *the outer circle* **(C)** (where the heart is a scarce resource, and where he may have to decide who, out of two or more potential recipients, will be given it). Or, if there is only one patient awaiting an organ, he will be operating within *the centre ring* **(A)**, with adequate resources at least in terms of organs. In this context Dr Smith's position within the Rings is entirely subject to the prevailing circumstances.

Perhaps Dr Smith wishes to transplant a kidney and has an adequate supply in his locality. But what he does not have is sufficient funding from his health authority or hospital to pay for support staff to provide a full service. And as a consequence patients are suffering, and in some cases dying, where they need not. In this case then he is actually standing in either **(C)** *(much rationing)* or **(B)** *(some rationing)* rings, but must—if he is a caring surgeon—be seeking to stand within the *centre ring* **(A)** *(adequate resources)*.

If he wishes to make progress—if he wishes to be creative with the various limits in which he finds himself—then Dr Smith may have to consider the extent of his role within limits other than resources. For instance, if he wishes to change the situation, he may have to reflect where he stands within the Rings expressed in terms of competence, and where he might conceivably move within these Rings.

At present he is a single consultant lacking staff. With the advantage of his professional status he can put some pressure on hospital management, but he can have no confidence that he can win his way. Perhaps he will have to move out from the centre to the second or third rings—perhaps the third ring—where he must work in a team with other consultants, or with other health workers. If he really wants to do something in these circumstances then Dr Smith must imagine himself standing within two sets of Rings at once. And he must consider where he should stand for the best within both sets of Rings.

Law

The law in relation to medical practice is a complex and uncertain affair (a very small part of this has been outlined in Chapter Two, where law was shown to contribute to the setting of norms in medicine). Given this fact, and given that change to a simpler system is not likely in the foreseeable future, it is a prudent doctor who seeks to recognise where he is positioned in the Rings expressed in terms of the law as it relates to medicine (Figure 5.4). Dependent upon his perceived position he may wish to alter his practice. For example, he may choose to practice 'defensive medicine' [78], and so be ultracautious whenever he pictures himself in the third Ring **(C)**, where the law is unpredictable.

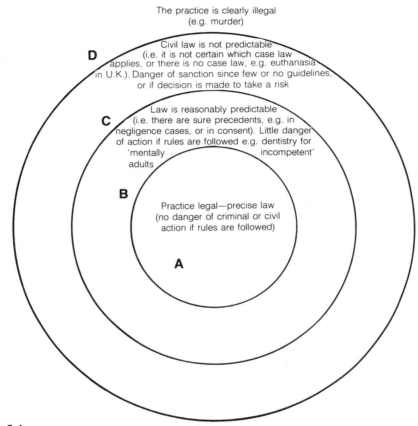

The practice is clearly illegal
(e.g. murder)

D Civil law is not predictable
(i.e. it is not certain which case law
applies, or there is no case law, e.g. euthanasia
in U.K.). Danger of sanction since few or no guidelines,
or if decision is made to take a risk

C Law is reasonably predictable
(i.e. there are sure precedents, e.g. in
negligence cases, or in consent). Little danger
of action if rules are followed e.g. dentistry for
'mentally   incompetent'
adults

B Practice legal—precise law
(no danger of criminal or civil
action if rules are followed)

A

Figure 5.4

The effect which *picturing* can have on practice is not unique to the Rings expressed in terms of law. For instance, when the Rings are expressed in terms of technical competence, dependent upon his perceived position, the doctor may decide to be decisively in charge (perhaps when the patient asks him sincerely to do so, when the patient is very ill or unconscious, or when the patient is deeply frightened) or clearly an agent for his patient, respecting the patient's beliefs and choices entirely. It is not the case that the doctor must always do what the patient wants—though he must always seek to create autonomy.

Within the Rings: an example in terms of law
Once again the focus of interest is the doctor's perception of his role. How should the doctor conceive of himself and his activity? How might this affect his actions? How might this *picturing* help define a limit around what the doctor might do?

Consider Dr Halsall, a general practitioner, who has been encouraged by his Family Practitioner Committee (who have in turn been urged by Government) to perform 'minor surgery' rather than refer his patients on for more expensive treatment in hospital. Where should he place himself within the Rings expressed in terms of law when a patient requests that he remove a verruca from her foot?

Should Dr Halsall picture himself in the *centre Ring* **(A)** (*where the law is clear*), or in another? If he thinks of himself as standing in the centre, by implication he believes that he need only worry about gaining the patient's consent for the operation, so as not to risk an accusation of battery. Given this, so long as he lives up to the standard set by the Bolam Test [79] he need not reflect further—particularly if he also sees himself standing within the centre of the Rings expressed in terms of technical competence and communication. But would Dr Halsall not be wise at least to place himself within the second Ring **(B)**, where he chances some danger of litigation if things go wrong? If he does so he might then take very great care that the area on which he has operated does not become infected, perhaps to the extent that he asks the patient back in daily so that a nurse might check the wound. Of course, in order to decide *this* question, he will need to picture himself within Rings expressed for other contents, particularly technical competence and resources.

Tension between different Rings   Since the Rings merely reflect considerations which must be taken into account in real-life decision-making it is often the case that, although a doctor may wish to place himself at certain points within Rings expressed for different contents, he will not be able to stand where he wants simultaneously in each Ring. Just as in real life doctors can wish to move in different directions at once, so there can be irreconcilable tensions between desired positions within the Rings in some contexts.

Take the case of Dr Greaves, who is consulted by a 57-year-old, retired, heavy smoking, 4 st overweight bus-driver with a history of angina, who says that he has had to stop and sit down for 15 minutes whilst walking because he was so short of breath, and felt some pain in his chest. Should Dr Greaves decide to sit plumb in the centre of the Rings expressed in terms of law and examine the man thoroughly, before referring him to the appropriate hospital consultant—or to Casualty—in order to attempt to prevent a possible heart attack? If he does this then he will be extremely prudent, but he will also use up valuable time. Alternatively, should Dr Greaves place himself at the centre of the Rings expressed in terms of resources, taking care to ensure that he has adequate time for each of his patients, whilst accepting the risk involved with a move into the third ring **(C)** of the Rings expressed in terms of law? If he decides to stand in **(C)** ring, if he decides to send the bus-driver away after a cursory examination, then he will have placed himself in danger of an accusation of negligence—of not meeting the accepted 'standard of care' of the competent general practitioner. What if the bus-driver actually suffers a heart attack?

Communication

The breadth of existing language, both general and technical, will persistently limit the extent of communication between doctors, and between doctors and patients. The study of language and communication is an enormously complex subject [80]. The aspect of the subject which is of most concern to doctors of medicine is usually the extent to which meaning is understood: *Does the patient have a clear picture of what I have said? Have I properly grasped what the patient is trying to describe to me?*

Consider pain. Pain is a word which can have great depth of meaning, but which is notoriously difficult to translate accurately. When a person is asked if she has a pain it is common for her to be asked its location and its severity. But if more detail is needed it is difficult, if not impossible, to tell if the intended meaning has been correctly conveyed. If she explains that the pain is 'stabbing' or 'deep' or 'intense' this may not be enough to establish a clear clinical picture without further investigation. And even if it is sufficient for a clinical assessment, none the less it may not put across a faithful representation of the pain. If a more detailed and extensive 'pain language' could be devised and put into common usage then the limits of language might stretch to allow deeper and more extensive communication between doctors and patients.

There are other examples in medicine of the way in which the limit on what may be communicated can expand. For instance, the language of psychiatry develops regularly [81]. And as new technology is invented (for example, 'body scanning' by 'magnetic resonance'), so new words and uses of language become necessary to describe the images produced. Equally, the limits may shrink. Some commentators [82] have

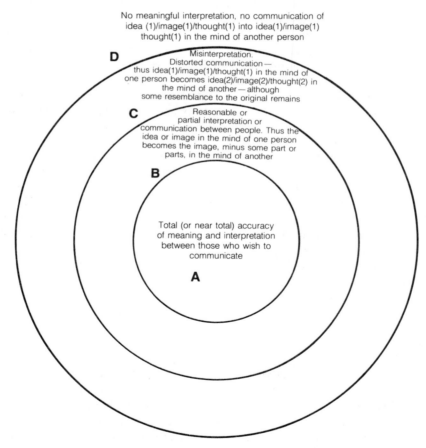

No meaningful interpretation, no communication of idea (1)/image(1)/thought(1) into idea(1)/image(1) thought(1) in the mind of another person

D

Misinterpretation. Distorted communication — thus idea(1)/image(1)/thought(1) in the mind of one person becomes idea(2)/image(2)/thought(2) in the mind of another — although some resemblance to the original remains

C

Reasonable or partial interpretation or communication between people. Thus the idea or image in the mind of one person becomes the image, minus some part or parts, in the mind of another

B

Total (or near total) accuracy of meaning and interpretation between those who wish to communicate

A

Figure 5.5

argued that this process occurred in the 1960s when 'reductionist science'* enjoyed its heyday. During this era words and phrases such as 'holistic', 'spiritual healing' and 'person-centred' were held by some clinicians to be empty—to be simply meaningless.

Figure 5.5 suggests one way of representing levels of communication in terms of the Rings of Uncertainty. The wording used considers language in the sense of *shared meaning between people who wish to communicate.*

This is only one possible formulation of the Rings expressed in terms of language and communication. The simple model cannot, without overstretching credibility and coherence, accommodate all possibilities†. However, this scheme will suffice for the most common difficulties associated with language use. It is not uncommon to underestimate the extent of these difficulties. The levels of language and communication are an important inclusion within the Rings of Uncertainty.

For example, whether using technical language or common language, it is frequently unclear whether full comprehension has occurred. It is well known that the use of technical terms—without fully explicit explanation—can generate unfortunate confusion. The word 'ethics', for instance, has a rich variety of meaning dependent upon who is speaking it and who is interpreting it. For some 'ethics' means 'a personal code of behaviour' and for others 'rules governing society'. And while the word 'therapy' may imply a neutral or enabling activity for most therapists, for some patients the word can carry with it connotations of blame and punishment. Some patients assume that they are literally responsible for their own illness, and see therapy as a form of penance—'I would not need therapy had I been a better person'. If what is meant is not specified clearly then some misunderstanding is probable.

Misunderstandings can occur as the result of the under-elaboration of fact (for example, 'go to bed and take bed-rest' might imply one day or one week of confinement); misperception of emphasis (for example, 'this operation has some risk, like all operations' might mean one thing to the doctor and quite another to the patient not least because it is the patient who must undergo the operation and the doctor who must perform or observe it); misinterpretation through ambiguity (for example, the words 'safe', 'cancer' and 'love' have a range of legitimate meanings). A good doctor must be careful that comprehension is as accurate as possible. Thus, for a doctor to attempt constantly to picture her position within the Rings expressed in this way can be a valuable exercise.

Although the Rings are not intended primarily for reference in urgent situations, but for times when quieter reflection is possible, this use of the imagination can be helpful during some consultations. In those meetings between doctors and patients which are especially fraught the level of understanding can change dependent upon the subject area and the depth to which it is being explained, and also dependent upon the effect of the information that is being communicated.

Reductionism is the belief that the way to understand more about nature is to gain knowledge about ever smaller parts of it. Thus it might be held that more can be learnt about disease through biochemistry than through social research.
†Equally this is one simple model of communication among the many which can be found in work in the philosophy of language. No attempt is made here to deal with its philosophical difficulties—for instance, how does one actually check that idea (1) remains idea (1) or has become idea (3)?

It is common for some news to have a dramatic effect on the level at which communication is possible. To take one example, it may be that in a communication between a doctor and patient who are from similar backgrounds (e.g. they are both professionals, both white, both men, both middle-class, both in their fifties) and are both articulate about the results of exploratory tests, the communication takes place entirely within either Rings **(A)** or **(B)**, until a certain point is reached in the conversation. Having explained the background to the tests, and having imparted some key factual information about the test process, when the doctor announces 'I'm afraid that the results show that you have an advanced malignancy—in other words, I'm sorry, you have cancer', suddenly the consultation leaps to levels **(C)** or **(D)**. Both the doctor and patient now exist in an area of heightened uncertainty.

While a person is shocked any attempt at communication is likely to be less meaningful. The rings can be a valuable reminder of the need to adapt one's work to a new set of circumstances.

In addition, the fact that the level of communication has changed may affect the position of the doctor within the Rings expressed in other terms. For example, movement may be necessary within the Rings expressed in terms of resources since more time may need to be spent. Similarly, since shock can adversely affect the reasoning process, a fresh positioning within the Rings expressed in terms of law and ethics might be necessary if the question of informed consent arises. If there is a serious problem of communication it may be that the Rings expressed in these terms assume the highest significance—if only temporarily.

This latest expression of the Rings leads the inquiry into the range and extent of limits to medicine into yet deeper complexity. It is now possible for the doctor who wishes to gain a clearer insight into the legitimate limits of his role, to picture himself standing within the Rings of Uncertainty expressed in terms of *competence, resources, law* and *communication*. Intriguingly, the doctor might conceive of himself standing at a different level for each expression of the Rings, and he might notice pulls and tensions if he conceives of his position within the Rings contrary to what reality will allow. However, although this model is potentially illuminating, the picture is in danger of becoming more confused than if the Rings had not been created. Some way of simplification, and of offering more exact guidance, is required. But before this is put forward it is important to notice that a crucial difference becomes apparent when an attempt is made to express the Rings in terms of levels of Ethics. Whereas it is possible to offer acceptable, albeit simplistic, terminology to express the Rings in terms of other categories, in the case of ethics this is far more difficult, if not impossible.

Ethics

There are two immediate difficulties encountered when an attempt is made to express the Rings in terms of ethics (Figure 5.6). Firstly, the labels seem so open to interpretation that they seem able to cover any conceivable intervention. Secondly, where one person chooses to place himself, or to imagine himself standing, may not be the place another person would put him for the same intervention. And in terms of the wording of the levels of ethics there seems to be no definitive way to resolve such a disagreement. To see ethics in such a simplistic way is actually a *category mistake*.

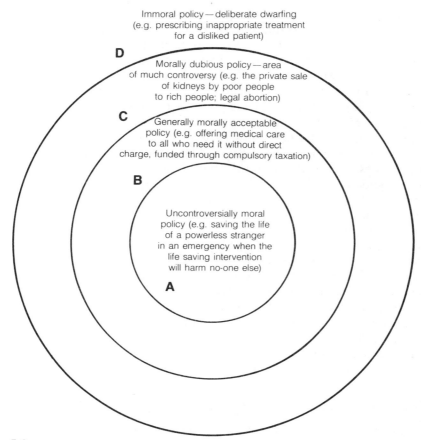

Immoral policy—deliberate dwarfing
(e.g. prescribing inappropriate treatment
for a disliked patient)

D

Morally dubious policy—area
of much controversy (e.g. the private sale
of kidneys by poor people
to rich people; legal abortion)

C

Generally morally acceptable
policy (e.g. offering medical care
to all who need it without direct
charge, funded through compulsory taxation)

B

Uncontroversially moral
policy (e.g. saving the life
of a powerless stranger
in an emergency when the
life saving intervention
will harm no-one else)

A

Figure 5.6

Consider Dr White, a general practitioner, reflecting upon what advice (or practical device) to offer Joanne who has come to see him with a request for a prescription for the contraceptive pill.

Joanne is just 15. She is categorised by those who find such classification useful as *lower working class*, and she has a strong accent and use of English peculiar to her locality. Dr White recognises that he has a problem which might best be understood in terms of ethics. Dr White also recognises that he could usefully visualise himself as standing within the Rings of Uncertainty translated in other ways. For example, he might choose to express them in terms of language and communication. Alternatively he might choose to express the Rings in terms of law—choosing to focus on the legal controversy which surrounded the Gillick case [83, 84]. However, Dr White decides that on balance his best option is to imagine himself standing within the Rings expressed in terms of ethics.

Dr White has not been confronted with a case such as this previously, but he is inclined towards any policy which helps other people and which respects their wishes. Consequently, as Joanne begins to blurt out that she wants the Pill, his basic instinct is to talk it through with her, and then, all being well, to prescribe the most appropriate drug. Dr White decides to clarify his position—because he knows that his instinct would not be shared by all doctors and suspects that it might be important to analyse his intuitive decision. But, as he conjures up his mental picture of a series of rings and tries to see himself within them, the image is confusing. He can see himself (and can imagine others placing him) within more than one circle.

Dr White is unsure whether to imagine himself in the second or third rings (the second indicates a generally acceptable policy, while the third designates a morally dubious policy—an area of much controversy). And further he is aware that there are those who would argue—vehemently in some cases—that by considering prescribing an oral contraceptive to a sexually active girl under the age of consent he is standing in area **(D)** (Mrs Gillick has taken this line). Equally, he recognises that there are some who would say that he is standing in Circle **(A)** (people in the Women's Rights Movement would usually take this view).

Clearly there is a peculiarity when the Rings are given meaning in terms of ethics: it is highly improbable that there will ever be consensus about the correct position for Dr White within these Rings, although if the Rings are expressed in terms of law or resources then such permanent controversy will not persist since Dr White's actual or potential position will essentially be a question of empirical verification. For instance, the current law is that doctors can prescribe the pill to under-age girls of sufficient maturity, but they must make efforts to encourage each girl to inform her parents or guardians [85]. And there are adequate supplies of the Pill, so there is no problem of resource in this case. But ethics lies within the realm of value judgement, and so is not as suitable as other subjects for presentation in the form of Rings. However, ethics is far from being 'just opinion', as is demonstrated in later chapters.

The limits to medicine—from insight to guidance

Up to this point it is fair to say that all that has been demonstrated is that in whatever dimension—clinical or non-clinical—medical decision-making is almost always complicated. But it is not the task of a philosophical work merely to describe what is already well known. Clarification, explanation, and practical assistance should also be expected. In order to offer practical guidance a model must be reasonably concise. It is too much to expect a doctor to retain five (or possibly more) images of Rings in her mind, and then to judge accurately what her role ought to be. The model currently offered requires further development.

Step Three

It is possible to simplify the Rings of Uncertainty by making use of only one set of Rings divided up into various segments (Figure 5.7). Such an image begins to offer more help to doctors who wish to understand the various factors which shape and limit medical practice.

Step Four

Making use of the single set of Rings, it is suggested that during the process of conceiving—during the process of *picturing* his position—a doctor experiments, placing

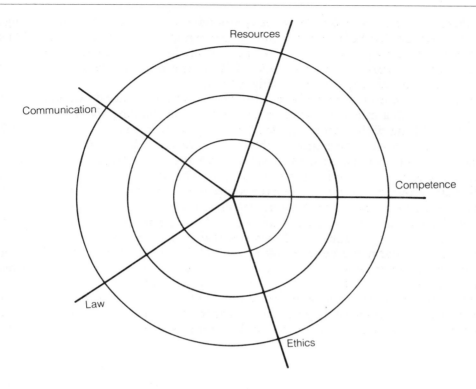

Figure 5.7

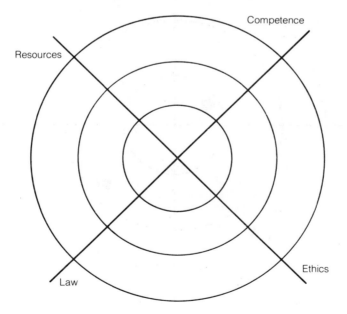

Figure 5.8

markers in what he considers to be the appropriate sections of the segmented rings. He may decide that he does not require every segment during this process. Thus, it may be that for a particular problem, a doctor thinks that the main considerations are *resources, competence, law* and *ethics*, and so chooses to divide up the Rings of Uncertainty in the way illustrated (Figure 5.8).

Perhaps the doctor is a general practitioner who needs to decide whether or not to proceed with a minor operation in his surgery. On thinking about it, using one segmented Ring with markers, he may come up with an image as in Figure 5.9.

This image is a representation of the doctor's decision. In order to arrive at the image, the doctor will have had to consider each of the categories. The image conveys the end-product of the decision-making process. The doctor has decided that he has adequate resources—he has the correct equipment, time and staff support. But in terms of technical competence he must collaborate with others; in this case he would need to ask detailed advice from a colleague who is a consultant surgeon. In terms of ethics his policy is dubious. He worries that it is a form of cost-cutting which involves risk, and that a better result might well be obtained in a hospital setting. In terms of law he believes that he runs some risk of litigation, primarily because of his position within the technical competence segment.

On balance the doctor decides not to carry out minor surgery. But his decision was made in a remarkably imprecise manner. It would be possible, but very cumbersome, to translate the decision-making process into a series of hypotheses and

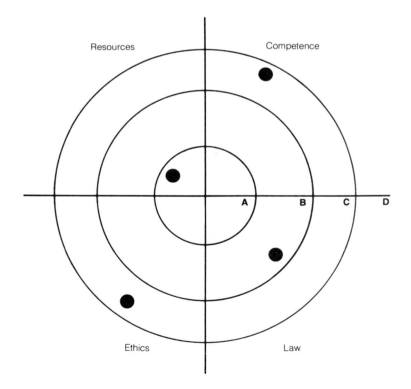

Figure 5.9

tests. For example, the doctor might begin by forming the hypothesis, *If I operate in my surgery, I run no extraordinary risk*. He might then express the possible risks in terms of the categories he has selected, and assess these separately, perhaps arriving at different conclusions for law and ethics. At a later point in his deliberation he might test the hypothesis, *By seeking the advice of a specialist surgeon, I minimise the risk of litigation if the operation is not a success*. But this would be only one among many hypotheses he would need to test.

Naturally such exhaustive hypothesis generation and testing is rarely if ever undertaken in the clinical context. Judging and reasoning is a far more fluid and agile human process. Fortunately it is possible to add more precision to the model. In this way it is possible to enhance the deliberations of doctors who wish to decide the most desirable form for a particular medical intervention. This method does not unduly distort the process of judging, nor does it corrupt an essentially qualitative process with artificial weightings.

Step Five

A key dictum

It will be obvious to all doctors that if their imaginative introspection displays them standing entirely outside the Rings of Uncertainty then they ought not intervene. This is a *clear practical limit to medicine*. For instance, if the potential intervention is believed to be immoral, illegal, and beyond communication, and the doctor has no resources for it and is incompetent, then only a fool would do it. Indeed, if the doctor is standing outside the Rings for any segment it is highly unlikely that he should act on a policy which places him in such a position.

It is possible to derive a key dictum from this that *if a doctor's image shows him standing outside the Rings for any segment then this is a very strong indication that a limit to medicine has been reached. Unless the circumstances are exceptional, the doctor should not proceed.*

However, there may be exceptional circumstances. It may be that for some segments at least, to stand beyond the Rings will not necessarily require the abandonment of the project. For instance, just because an action is said to be illegal it is not always out of the question, especially if the doctor is simultaneously standing within the Rings expressed for ethics. Euthanasia is a good example of this.

As a general guide it can be said that *the further towards the edges of the Rings a doctor sees herself actually or potentially standing, the more reason she has to question the wisdom of her situation or plan*. However, this guideline is still too general to be of much practical use. What if the doctor has divided her Ring of Uncertainty into four segments and conceives of herself as standing in the centre for two segments and at the edges of the outer ring for the other two segments? How is she to assess her most appropriate role in these circumstances?

One option open to her is to embark on a process of detailed moral reasoning to assess the wisdom of her proposed intervention (so overriding the Rings). But this requires a sophisticated training and an extensive knowledge of moral philosophy which she is unlikely to have. Happily, it is yet possible to discover more precision using only the Rings.

Step Six

The Rings cannot be used abstractly. They make sense only with the addition of the content of the situation, and the circumstances of the particular doctor. Dependent upon content and circumstance the importance of any segment will vary. Taking note of this, further life can be breathed into the Rings by allowing the segments to be *movable*, not to have a fixed area but to have a changeable size. The lines dividing the segments can be imagined to pivot around the centre-point of the Rings, and to be alterable, like the hands on a carriage-clock.

Thus it may be that if a doctor decides, for a particular case, that there are three key considerations (e.g. *technical competence, resources* and *law*) he will not be restricted to a static model of this type (Figure 5.10).

Instead he will be able to reflect upon his decision by according each consideration a *relative* importance (Figure 5.11).

By altering the segments in such a way the doctor indicates a belief that the extent of his medical skill and knowledge is the main concern in this case. His decision about where he stands within the Rings expressed in terms of competence will have a crucial influence on the form of his practice.

This flexibility, this mobility, is not of overriding importance for the individual doctor faced with an imminent decision. For if the doctor sees himself outside the Rings expressed in terms of *law* or *resources*, however small the area of the segment, this remains a strong indication that the potential intervention should not go ahead. The flexibility takes on a greater importance when the idea of the Rings is applied to an analysis of the shape of medical education as a whole (see Chapter Seven).

Scoring and quantification

The Rings of Uncertainty are designed primarily as conceptual guidelines, not to provide rigid, quantifiable rulings. However, it might be that individual doctors will wish to invent a personal scoring system, particularly if their specialisation is such that they tend to conceive of most or all of their markers as placed neither in the centre of the Rings nor on the outside whenever they have to make a decision. It may be that for some doctors a system of numbers could prove decisive in borderline instances where the doctor must choose whether or not to go forward with a particular form of intervention. For example, as one means of orientation amongst others, a doctor might decide to score the centre of the Rings as four, the next ring as three, the outer ring as two, and the surrounding area as zero. She might decide that she will add up the scores for each ring, divide by the number of segments, and accept a cut-off point of say, less than three, as a guide that she should not proceed. If she chooses a lower cut-off point, then she will be choosing to take greater risks, but may find other benefits along the way.

To act as a reasonable guide the Rings must be precise enough to generate some sort of score, but flexible enough to reflect the fact that deliberation about medical intervention frequently transcends crude counting. The Rings offer the possibility for doctors to invent a basic scoring system to set limits to their activity. But this system must always take into account the vagaries of life—the aspects of care which cannot be effectively modelled. For instance, dependent upon the context it may

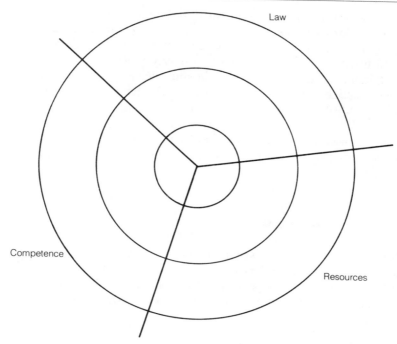

Figure 5.10

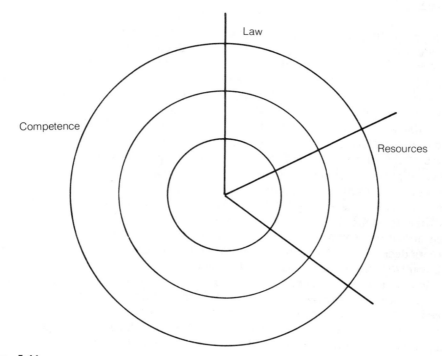

Figure 5.11

not always be a disadvantage for a doctor to be standing in the outer circles for the Rings expressed for *competence*, *ethics* and *law*. So to score less than three, or less than whatever other figure is selected by the doctor, need not imply that a halt must be called. In order for a doctor to assess properly whether or not to intervene he must have thought through his priorities, he must be clear about the main theoretical drives of his practice. The primary purpose of the Rings of Uncertainty is not to offer a dubious 'ideal solution' to the question, '*At what point, for how long, and in what way should I intervene?*'. The Rings are meant to move doctors to the point where they recognise that it is essential to have a coherent opinion about the importance of their work, and also to offer a logical starting point for the development of such a rationale.

A further educational use

The scoring system could be used to review the past performances of doctors, as a learning experience, to enable them to consider whether or not they should have intervened in the way that they chose to. Or if this were to prove too threatening the scoring system could be used to assess hypothetical doctors in invented cases.

A conclusion

One clear conclusion to emerge so far from this account of the Rings is that, in order to weigh the many variables adequately, the doctor must use a rich model of medicine—she must be operating with a wide theory about the purpose of medical work. By definition, if she recognises the need to reflect upon ethics, communication, the law, resources and her own level of competence she will realise that the best medicine must involve both clinical and non-clinical judgement. The doctor who believes that all he must do in order to practise adequately is to be clinically competent is denying most of the reality of the care of human beings.

In truth, in order to use the Rings properly, it is necessary for doctors to possess well-reasoned views about why their work is valuable, about why health-care is substantially different from accountancy or legal work (both of which are professions which work closely with people). Presently, many doctors hold only implicit views about the importance of health care. Such doctors tend to defend 'the health service' against attack more with rhetoric than reason. But this situation is not inevitable. If doctors decide that it is useful to employ this simple model then, in order to use it to advantage, they must consider what their overall priorities are, or should be. Some doctors may well accept the theory of *health as foundations* since at least part of this framework already seems to be present in the political writings of many doctors.

In order to take this framework further still, two more elements need to be added. These are the *Autonomy Test* and *full moral reasoning*. But such advances must be developed slowly. In order for doctors to experiment with the Rings of Uncertainty the following exercise is suggested. It should be read as an essential part of Chapter Five.

Exercise Four

Using the Rings of Uncertainty fully expressed

Consider this difficult scenario in medicine, and imagine how a doctor might deal with it by employing the Rings as an aid to his deliberation.

Dr Wilson is a consultant paediatrician facing an unpleasant dilemma. He is responsible for the care of a severely handicapped neonate—a week-old child. The baby has an inoperable condition but, with prolonged intensive care stands a 50% chance of surviving, at least for a few years. However, it is likely that his distress—both mental and physical will be so great that many people would not judge his life to be worth living. The child's parents are extremely distressed. They are both Catholic.

Dr Wilson, as a general rule, concerns himself only with the patients who are actually in his care. He believes that he cannot be expected to consider potential patients as well—even though because of lack of facilities he may have to turn away some who have better chances than his current patients. The doctor is accustomed to dramatic medicine, where he will often make 'heroic' interventions. He believes that 'death with dignity' is a crucial concept for his particular branch of medicine. And further that 'letting die' is fundamentally different from 'killing', and is preferable by far.

However, Dr Wilson is a thoughtful doctor, inclined to reassess his position periodically. He decides that his present dilemma—which is whether or not to continue intensive care for the baby—provides a good opportunity for a re-examination of his motives and his role. He decides to picture himself within the Rings of Uncertainty.

The primary issue here is not 'What should I do?', although this is a question that he must answer, but 'What is my proper role here? To what extent ought I intervene in this situation? To what extent am I equipped to undertake the various options?'

The Rings expressed

Dr Wilson considers that he needs to use all the available segments: *competence*, *resources*, *law*, *communication* and *ethics*. Thus he has an initial picture of the Rings as shown in Figure 5.12.

Dr Wilson is not sure, without thinking the problem through, how large each segment should be—so he decides to leave them roughly equal. Even the relative importance of the elements of the problem is uncertain at this stage.

How can Dr Wilson perceive of his position? How is he to determine his proper role in this case? What must limit his medical practice?

Clearly there are several considerations, several potential limits, and several possible courses of action in play in this case. Not all of the options will be of the same merit, but more than one might be chosen by 'the reasonable doctor'. Dr Wilson begins to explore the Rings. Logically enough he begins in the *competence* segment. Now, if Dr Wilson conceives of himself standing outside the Rings—where he has no special skill or knowledge—he should stop his deliberation at this initial thought. If he is not competent to make the decision about whether to cease intensive care, then he should pass the problem over to someone else, or to a team of people. Perhaps a nurse, or a priest, or a philosopher or the parents will be better equipped to make the best decision.

continued on next page

continued

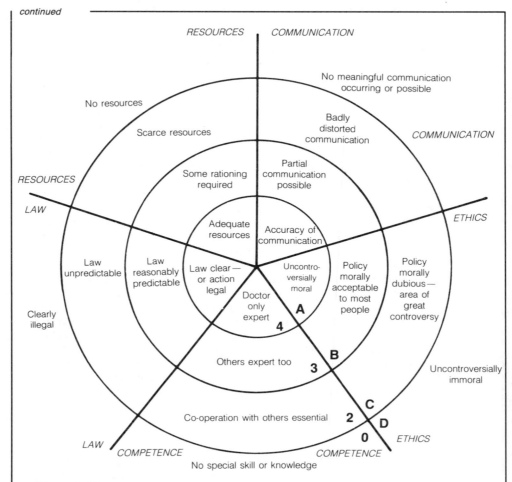

Figure 5.12

In fact Dr Wilson is not so unassuming. Tentatively, he places himself within the second circle from the centre **(B)**, thus acknowledging that others are expert too. But he is careful not to annul his option to assert his power, if he thinks it necessary. By picturing himself as standing in this part circle for the Rings expressed in terms of technical competence Dr Wilson has retained the right to continue to reflect about his role. He does not believe that, in this case, his less-than-perfect competence should limit his medical activity. He may not be right, however. He is deliberating only with himself. He may face a tougher test to establish his claim to a role in conversation with others.

He does worry about the law. He is profoundly aware of the Arthur case [86] and of Re B[87]. As he understands the law, if he were to kill the baby by poisoning him, then he might run the risk of a charge of murder. If he intends active euthanasia, then the law might well act as a serious restriction. But this is not his intention.

Dr Wilson has long held the belief that to discontinue treatment is not a positive act. For him (although not everyone shares this view [88]) not doing something is

continued on next page

continued

not 'morally equivalent' to doing something. If there were no medical knowledge the child would not be alive in any case. Not to treat is natural. Doctors are not 'Gods'. Sometimes it is better to 'let nature take its course'. Dr Wilson is familiar with many precedents for this (he has made similar interventions in the past, and he is reassured that Dr Arthur was not found guilty). However, he recognises that there is some risk of legal action, and so places himself in the second innermost Ring **(B)**, since he regards the law as only reasonably predictable.

He does appreciate that he ought to involve the parents if at all possible, to ascertain what they wish. However, there are tremendous problems of communication. Both are Catholic and regard life as sacred, but both are also acutely aware of the horrifying condition of their baby. They are crying, grieving already, and their competence to reason calmly is obviously diminished. In addition, it is hard for all concerned to discuss ending the life of the baby. Consequently Dr Wilson decides to close up the communication segment, making it comparatively small—he doesn't regard it as particularly important. He places himself in the outer circle of the small segment **(C)**, believing that communication, if it is possible at all, will inevitably be badly distorted. Dr Wilson believes further that since he has considered the possibility that there are others (the parents) of equal expertise to him, and he has found them to be temporarily incapacitated, he must now see himself as standing within the centre circle for technical competence **(A)**, moving inwards one circle. Only he is expert at this decision. He feels that if he decides to discontinue treatment (which is his inclination) then it will be important to ensure that the parents do not suffer guilt—he will remove this future burden from them.

At this point he would certainly face a strong challenge from other quarters. Dr Wilson does not have access to some 'moral truth'. It is very possible that a stronger justification might be advanced for an alternative policy. However, the purpose of describing a doctor reflecting upon his position within the Rings of Uncertainty is to display the working of the process rather than to advance a deep and perfect moral argument.

As far as resources are concerned, these are adequate. He is within the centre circle for this segment—he has time, staff, equipment, and finance. Treatment is available for the child, if it is considered appropriate. However, afterwards, if the baby survives, he will continue to need expensive care. Even later there will be a significant demand on state resources to maintain and support the infant.

Dr Wilson looks at the image he has produced and recognises that he has arrived at a decision. Dr Wilson's image of the Rings of Uncertainty looks like Figure 5.13.

According to his personal scoring system Dr Wilson feels that he should—in the best interest of the child and her parents—discontinue intensive care. He thinks that to discontinue the treatment would be acceptable to most people, especially if they could see the mutilation and suffering. He recognises that he does not know this for sure, and he is aware that to let the child die will neither be purely immoral nor moral. He knows that whatever decision he takes will be contentious, but he prefers to think that most reasonable people would side with his opinion.

He scores 16 divided by 5, an average score of over 3. He believes he has a role. He is operating within a variety of uncertainties. In addition to his uncertainties of interpretation, of ethics, and of self, he does not know what will happen to the child if therapy is discontinued. Dr Wilson is clear, however, that he is operating within the limits of medicine. 'Who else', he asks, 'could take such a decision?'

continued on next page

continued

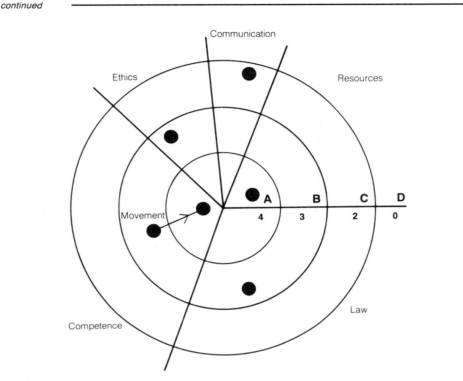

Figure 5.13

Other people might place Dr Wilson in different circles, and set the segments to different sizes. However, because Dr Wilson has produced a clear, graphic image, because he has made his deliberation about the extent of his role overt and explicit, the use of the Rings at least allows meaningful conversation to start.

The case of the badly handicapped neonate is not one which can have a happy solution. Whatever the decision, there will be tragedy. A more complete ethical analysis would involve a detailed consideration of the range of cost and benefits, a discussion of the doctor's duty and priorities, and an assessment of the severity of the various potential harms (or dwarfings) with a view to minimising them.

Do you agree with Dr Wilson's use of the Rings?

Can the Rings Really Help Limit Medicine in a Useful Way?

The following criticism might be made of the Rings.

This modelling—this glossy description—is pretty enough, but it is no better a way of arriving at decisions than any other commonsense way based on experience. It may be true that most doctors find it difficult to decide where their role begins and ends—'To what extent should I actively try to prevent problems, and to what extent should I involve myself in helping those people who come to me, or even those who don't?'

But merely to illustrate the conundrum in terms of Rings does not move the problem nearer a solution. There are two specific areas where the Rings are just of no help at all:

(1)   Doctors have to make many judgements in medicine, many of which they make intuitively, or at least not overtly. Doctors recognise that they make these judgements, and do not need them further highlighting. The Rings are patronising, and in any case simply replace one implicit judgement with another. The Rings are of no help to the doctor who has to decide the size of each segment.

(2)   It is said that the point of the Rings is to help the doctor reach a careful decision about whether to intervene or not—or whether to continue to intervene. And if he decides to intervene, to help him judge which areas for intervention, and which ways of intervention are most appropriate. However, everything still rests upon the doctor's opinion. If she decides that she must help a patient apply for housing benefit, or if she decides that she must devote all her energies towards a campaign against a Government White Paper on the Health Service, then that is for her to judge. There can be no other arbiter of this decision, certainly not the Rings of Uncertainty.

Response to these criticisms

It is true to say that doctors have to interpret the area and extent of the uncertainties with which they have to deal. A doctor could not act without making some judgement of this kind. However not every doctor reasons explicitly. Many believe that such decisions about how to proceed can be based only on precedent and intuition. Consequently their judging process is not open to test or debate. And at least some of those who do reason openly and in language about these issues do not do so as comprehensively as the Rings allow. At least by using the Rings to picture where he stands, to help him decide whether to go ahead or not, the doctor must pay attention to the level of his technical competence, the state of the law, the morality of his proposed action, the degree of shared comprehension which exists, and the level of resources he has available. The Rings help draw attention to these matters, which might otherwise be insufficiently noticed. And they can produce firm answers to the question 'What should the limit of my role be in this case?'

It is not true that decisions about where a doctor's role can or should start and finish are entirely a matter of opinion. Disagreement will always exist between advocates of the various models of medicine about the type of intervention that a doctor ought to undertake in controversial, specific situations. Such disagreement is inevitable in the moral realm. However, the Rings are able to offer assistance in the process of objective judgement about some of the limits to medical intervention.

For instance, if the doctor who wishes to campaign against the White Paper 'Working for Patients' [89] conceives of herself standing within the Rings of Uncertainty expressed in terms of competence, resources and language, and then thinks honestly in each of these areas, she might picture herself scoring zero for technical competence (no experience of campaigning, no political education), two for resources (no access to word-processing or publishing facilities, very little personal time to devote to the task, no other people supporting her efforts locally), and two for communication (good knowledge of clinical language, but little skill in the use of rhetoric, or in selecting key points for presentation to the media). Given this picturing, it is clear that the proposed action ought not to take place, since it can do no good and might cause harm, whilst she might intervene positively elsewhere making use of her other talents.

Equally, if she pictures herself within the Rings when considering the possibility of helping a patient apply for housing benefit, and finds that she is in the centre circle for every segment (when the patient has tried every other avenue for help available locally) then, almost certainly, she ought to go ahead and help him.

The Rings can also be of help in more ambiguous circumstances. It may be that doctor's projected position within only one of the segments will help him to decide whether to proceed or not. Perhaps he will be in Rings (**C**) *or* (**B**) *for all segments other than that for the Rings expressed for ethics, and close to the centre for ethics. It may be this emphasis on the moral desirability of the proposed action that swings it, perhaps helping the doctor to decide to override considerable uncertainty about the legality of the proposal (for instance, he might be considering breaking a confidence in 'the public interest'). Or perhaps the doctor will picture himself standing at the centre of each segment expressed for every category except law, where he stands at zero. Perhaps here he will decide to obey the law, although having made use of the Rings he may do so with more reluctance than he might otherwise have felt.*

Review

It should be clear that foremost among all the considerations raised in this book the key issue for doctors is where to draw the line over their interventions. Whatever the particular circumstances of a consultation, or of some other health-care activity, the doctor (or indeed any health worker) must address the question, '*What should I do, and where should I stop?*' The stop point might be generated by limits of competence, ethics, law, or resources—or some subtle combination of these—but it must be generated. Other people's lives are too important for the doctor just to allow this to happen—to be controlled by events. The doctor must be able to be clear where the limit falls.

It is an essential part of the liberation of medicine proposed in this book that doctors must be able to interpret and *experiment* with the Rings to explore how they might work. Doctors ought to be as free as possible to explore the extent to which each doctor can be useful, and the point at which the doctor begins to diminish or dwarf. In other words, within the limits to medicine, doctors must be able to be as creative as possible.

In addition it is vital to appreciate that if working with the Rings is to be of any use to a doctor she must recognise that other health workers—nurses, receptionists, health educators, and patients—will each 'see' themselves within their own rings—and that the rings of other health workers may *clash*. Indeed the *picturings* of the various health workers may clash to such an extent that different workers may consider themselves to be operating within different limits.

This is a major implication for health care as a whole. It is explored in more detail in the final chapter. At this point it is important to note:

(1)   The presence of the Rings can provide a framework for conversation about the appropriate roles of all health carers, including patients.

(2) The presence of the Rings can provide a representation of the range of limits to health care, although they cannot give a comprehensive guide. Deeper ethical analysis is required for this purpose.
(3) By using the Rings, and arguing for fresh placings within the circles, health carers have a powerful vehicle to campaign for change in health care.

Arguing for change in health care by the use of the Rings

The use of the Rings alone is not sufficient to argue thoroughly for change in health care. It is a prerequisite of a decent argument that the person expressing it has thought through the priorities implied by the notion of *work for health*, and is able to provide a coherent justification for them. However, the Rings can be useful to highlight problems of role, and so can assist arguments for changes of role. For example, if a nurse wishes to gain an expanded role for herself and her profession then she might ask a doctor to create an image of the doctor's role in a proposed intervention, while at the same time the nurse creates her image for the same intervention. Naturally both parties will need to be honest since both will already have an idea about how both images will appear. But so long as both are frank, after the markers have been placed within the two sets of Rings of Uncertainty the Rings might then be superimposed to good effect.

In this way a striking picture of differences and similarities in potential role will be seen. The doctor and nurse will need to discuss what they mean for each of the categories, but given this clarification it will be possible for the nurse to argue (perhaps in terms of competence, or resource, or communication) that her role should expand. And equally possible for the doctor to do the same if she feels that care will be better for it.

This insight is expanded in the final chapter.

Exercise Five

Live or Let Die?: Uncertainty of Role

Consider an emotionally fraught disagreement between two adult children about the treatment of their dying mother.

The mother is in her eighties. She suffered a severe stroke two years previously which completely paralysed one side of her body. Between then and now the mother has been cared for full-time by her 48-year-old daughter. The son has a home in America, where he works as an engineer.

Now the mother has contracted pneumonia, and is semicomatose. On diagnosing the condition the doctor speaks to both the son and the daughter, outlining the options, which are: do nothing (in which case death is likely in days); treat with antibiotics at home (in which case the infection may clear, only to return shortly); to treat 'aggressively' in hospital (in which case the infection may be resisted for longer). The daughter, feeling that her mother is no longer 'properly alive', wishes nothing to be done. But the son wants 'everything possible' to be done to save his mother.

continued on next page

continued

The doctor counsels both son and daughter, who fail to reach agreement. The doctor then calls in key relatives, including the sister of the sick woman, who eventually persuade the son to concur with his sister to do nothing.

Setting aside discussion about the 'morality' of euthanasia, the central issue in this case concerns the role of the doctor. At present her clinical training equips her to diagnose the condition, and prescribe appropriate treatment. It does not, usually, equip her to counsel. And it certainly does not legitimise interventions beyond the treatment of disease, and certainly not into the lives of others who have no disease. It is fair to say, 'What else could she do in such a situation?' But it is also essential to recognise the need for clarification of the doctor's role—both in order to protect currently practising doctors, and to ensure that medical students can be trained most appropriately to deal with—and work within—their role and limits of intervention.

Thought play

Consider the limit of the doctor's role by the use of the Rings of Uncertainty fully expressed. Include any further background details you feel necessary—or imagine yourself to be the doctor in question tackling a similar case.

Exercise Six

Dealing with Dying

If this exercise is to be used for either a role play or a thought play then select a character.

The characters

Louise (a woman close to death from cancer)
Daniel (her son)
Dr Jonathan Cook (senior lecturer in oncology—cancer specialist)
Marianne (an SRN on Ward Twelve)

Louise

Louise is a widow of 48 first diagnosed as having breast cancer four years ago. She underwent a radical mastectomy followed by radiotherapy and a course of chemotherapy. Two years after her operation she was found to have a recurrence in her lymph node. Now a brain secondary has been confirmed. Louise has been admitted to Ward Twelve. This ward is often used to house terminally ill patients, although other people with cancers are also cared for here. Louise has been a patient on this ward three times before.

Louise has not been told explicitly by anyone that she has a brain secondary. However she feels prepared for death, but has not yet been able to talk about her

continued on next page

continued

mortality with anyone in her family other than her sister, with whom she has often stayed during the years of her illness. She told Dr Cook a few months ago that he was not to continue treating her to keep her alive when things had become just too hopeless.

It is almost Christmas, and the ward is plastered with tinsel, greeting cards and plastic images of Santa Claus. Christmas has a reassuring continuity which Louise thinks is nice. She feels surrounded by other Christmases. Images of her late husband, and a house full of excited young children expecting carloads of friends and relatives, pass through her mind. Louise feels as if she is in a daze, she is confused and lucid only at times. When she can make sense she seems to talk more as a little girl than a woman.

But this is some sort of defence, helped by her pain-killing drugs. She knows she is dying. She feels deeply tired, although when she occasionally becomes more alert she seems to reawaken. When this happens she expresses regret at her passivity, 'she doesn't know what came over her', and reasserts her determination to fight, to get better. Louise is a mixture of emotions, a cocktail of denial, resistance and acceptance.

When she accepts she can think only of a single wish, which she does not think she has the strength to fulfil. She wishes she could tell Daniel simply that she loves him.

Daniel

Daniel is 24, and the eldest of Louise's three children. By coincidence he lives close to the hospital where his mother is being treated, while his brother and sister live over 90 miles away. He feels he must somehow assume responsibility as the chief next-of-kin of his mother, and so he visits her every day.

Daniel feels that he is a disappointment to his mother. As a youth he was far more concerned to have a good time than to study or pursue any career ambition. But he is now in his second year at the local university where he is a mature student. It took a lot of work and self-control to get to university and he wishes that his mother would acknowledge his recent efforts. He believes (with justification) that his mother sees him as 'the bad sheep'—a bit of a waster.

He feels numb. He knows that his Mum must die soon, but cannot grasp this as a reality. He cannot imagine his mother dying, he cannot picture this as a possibility. Looking out of the window of the bus to the hospital each day the world seems more distant than before, as if he were an observer and not really taking part in any of it. During his visits the conversation is slow and sparse. Daniel and his mother talk about plants and pets, which are mutual interests, but nothing more important. He feels he would like to express *everything* he has ever felt for his mother: his anger, his hopes, his sorrow for hurting her, but he cannot even form the specific thought in his mind—'I want to tell her that I love her'. At the time when he is with her he closes in on himself.

Dr Jonathan Cook

Dr Cook is a senior doctor aged 50. He has vast experience of cancer treatment and prognosis, and of the medical care of the dying. He is a hard-working academic and a kind man. Dr Cook thinks of Louise as an exceptional patient. He believes that without her determination she would have been dead two years ago, but she is a

continued on next page

continued

fighter and he knows how important that is in cancer patients. Dr Cook is also fond of Louise. He is a similar age, and from a similar background to his patient. They have had some frank conversations during the treatment programme, but now he feels less able to be open.

He has not thought through the reasons why his attitude has changed, but has withdrawn rapidly from the relationship. He now keeps a 'professional distance' and is leaving virtually all the care to the nursing staff. He has, and still has everyday, the opportunity to tell her that she definitely has a brain tumour, and is approaching death. But he does not do it. Louise is now under the direct care of a more junior doctor, and Dr Cook feels that speaking to Louise is no longer his role. If the other doctor wishes to tell her then that is for him to decide.

Marianne

Marianne hates this ward. She finds it desperately stressful to have to nurse people who are dying and often in great distress. She has applied for a transfer to intensive care where there is at least as much stress, but where people do recover. Marianne has been nursing Louise for three weeks, and is truly torn by the experience. When Louise is lucid and talking of getting better and going home, Marianne feels very close to her. Louise has a very sweet nature which makes Marianne think of her own mother. When Louise is in decline, Marianne wishes that she wouldn't wake up.

Marianne has observed the relationship between Louise and her son, and she is familiar with the difficulties they are having with communication. She can see that they are exceptionally bad at it, and it upsets her.

Marianne is always cheerful on the surface, always the jolly nurse. Daniel scowls at her when he sees her. He thinks that, like the Christmas decor, her gaiety is quite inappropriate. Marianne doesn't understand this, and thinks that he is very unpleasant and rather an inadequate young man. Why doesn't he just hold his mother's hand?

Marianne is compassionate, and has spoken to the social worker to ask her to speak to Daniel. She doesn't feel able to speak to Daniel and Louise herself to try to encourage them to talk to resolve their relationship.

The situation

There is a crisis. Daniel has come for an afternoon visit. Louise is drowsy, but conscious. She is lying on her side, and she is breathing wheezily. She seems very warm to Daniel as he leans over her to whisper hello. She seems to smell of babies. As he moves to find a chair so that he can speak to his mother he notices that her saline drip has gone. First he is pleased, he feels a surge of hope. But then he thinks again, as he sits quiet and still. A middle-aged woman in the bed opposite catches his eye, and starts to talk to him.

"Its a shame, its a shame, it really is. She's not very old . . . neither are you. It's a shame. I know her well you know. We were in here together last year. Oh, . . . it really is a shame . . ."

What's she talking like this for? In fear Daniel jumps up, he runs to the desk and asks Marianne what's happening (he doesn't know her name). She says that she is not sure but that Dr Cook has said that Louise is not to be disturbed anymore, and that she is not to have any more medication.

continued on next page

continued

"Where is he? I want to see him. Please." Daniel is first polite, then he begins to shout. "Where is that bloody doctor? I want him here now. He doesn't know what he is doing. Please. I'm not leaving until he comes. Please get him here. Get him here." Becoming increasingly agitated, Daniel leans over the desk and begins to push notes and files to the floor.

Role play/thought play

(1) Imagine the situation up to now from the point of view of your selected character. Try hard to imagine the situation from the points of view of other characters.
(2) Now act out in your imagination what happens next, playing the part of your selected character. Imagine the situation from the points of view of other characters.
(3) If in a class with others, act out the situation as a role play.

What are the main implications of this situation? What should the role of the doctor and the nurse be? What skills might they need?

Using the Rings fully expressed

(1) Select a character (either Dr Cook or Marianne).
(2) Decide on a policy—decide what to do next.
(3) Using the Rings fully expressed (see Figure 5.12) place markers/picture yourself within the Rings. If you like, calculate the level of risk of the policy. Remember that you can alter the size of the segments.

Examples: Marianne might decide to expel Daniel from the ward. She may attempt to do this herself.
Dr Cook might agree to recommence treatment.
Dr Cook and Marianne might decide to call on others—perhaps including Social Work staff—for help.

Chapter Six

The Autonomy Test

Introduction

In the previous chapter the Rings of Uncertainty were offered as a conceptual tool to enable doctors to begin to think more deeply about their roles and the limits to their power. The description of the Rings was also presented as a means of progressing the general argument of the book. During this process of elucidation it became clear that while it is generally the case that the meaning of the content of each segment requires interpretation, it is particularly difficult to give unambiguous wording to the ethics segment.

In part this is a difficulty inherent in presenting any model intended to be both an overview and a guide—a tool to which the user can add new meaning if he wishes. But the wording of the ethics segment is strikingly inadequate. It is plainly unsatisfactory to suggest that a policy can be said to be more or less moral in proportion to its level of popularity. If this were to be the case then judgements of morality would alter dependent upon swings of mood and attitude within populations. No moral philosopher would be happy to allow this to stand as a final ruling on the nature of ethics: Hitler's policies did not become less moral as the German people turned against them when defeat in the Second World War became increasingly probable. It is wrong to think that the wording of the ethics segment can suffice as anything other than a vague guideline. In fact moral deliberation is an extraordinarily complex process if it is done thoroughly, and such a process cannot be properly represented in any simple way [90].

However, in a practical book—especially in a practical book which seeks to suggest meaningful limits to medical activity—it is important to offer clear guidelines. One such a guideline is given in the *Autonomy Test* outlined in this chapter. *Like all guidelines in ethics, it is not suggested as a binding rule, nor is it necessarily appropriate to all cases that doctors might encounter.* But it is useful in certain contexts. For instance on occasions the *Autonomy Test* can act as a reminder to a doctor that he may be committing the *category mistake,* and should think again about his proposed intervention.

The Importance of Autonomy

There are several ethical principles which might have a claim to be the primary guiding force in health care. *'Being just'*, *'not doing harm'*, and *'doing positive good at all times'* are all candidates [91]. At times, dependent upon the context, each of these can assume a temporary priority, sometimes overriding the 'autonomy of individuals'—at least where autonomy means an 'individual getting what she wishes'. For example, in cases where a desired resource—perhaps a particularly expensive drug treatment—is scarce not all 'autonomy claims' can be met: not everybody can get what he wants.

It must be said that, in part, to select one idea as ultimately of more importance than any other carries with it an element of prejudice—it depends to some extent upon personal choice and values. However, it is possible to justify the selection of autonomy as the most important notion in health care in several plausible ways. Indeed, to say of autonomy that it has no importance in health care is simply a contradiction in terms in any meaningful account of health and health work.

Ways of justifying the view that the notion of autonomy is basic to health care

There are at least four pointers which indicate the importance of autonomy in general. These are that:

(1)   The law regards consent as an essential requirement in any legitimate health care intervention which involves touching. Without consent such an intervention will be either a civil or a criminal offence. In order for a person to consent to an operation he must have sufficient knowledge and grasp of what is proposed in order to understand the implications. To put this another way, his level of *autonomy* must be of a degree sufficient to give him control over the decision about whether to go ahead or not.

(2)   There is no difference in kind, only difference of *degree*, between the problem of disease and other problems of life. All problems tend to affect an individual's level of autonomy—when a person has a problem, by definition that person's autonomy is lessened, at least in the area of her life where the problem exists. Because disease is not radically different from other problems doctors are under no special obligation to fight it. The justification for work against disease must always refer to the creation of autonomy as a fundamental priority.

(3)   Medicine as work for health must work to liberate enhancing human potentials. Medicine as health work can diminish only when this diminishing avoids worse harms. This enhancement is ultimately, necessarily, the enhancement of autonomy.

(4)   If autonomy is taken to be a priority then the autonomy referred to cannot be only physical autonomy, unless a quite arbitrary distinction is to be made between the physical and mental mobility of a person. Work to create physical autonomy should not have the effect of impeding mental autonomy if the possibility of such autonomy exists in a person.

These justifications make full sense only when a basic distinction is made within the broad notion of autonomy. Essentially this distinction is between Understanding A—*autonomy as being able to do*—and Understanding B—*autonomy as being able to have one's expressed wants*. This distinction is developed during the course of this chapter.

Below are brief summaries of the four possible ways to justify the view that autonomy ought to be the fundamental value in health care.

Consent to treatment regarded by law as an essential requirement—consent requires a certain level of autonomy—certain *conditions* necessary.

Disease needs to be perceived to be a problem to count as a problem. No objective cut off between 'diseases' and other problems of life.

AUTONOMY

Medicine works to free—to liberate impeded potentials—not to diminish.

The mental life of a person is, at least, equally as important as his physical life—one should not create autonomy as physical doing at the expense of autonomy as thinking.

Autonomy may be basic to health care but it is not the only inspiration. In complicated situations a full process of deliberation must occur, where a range of factors are considered. However, no genuine health work can take place which makes no attempt to raise levels of autonomy [92].

The Richness of Autonomy

It is crucial to the argument being developed in this book to demonstrate the richness of the notion of autonomy. This richness is invariably overlooked by the lay writings of doctors on what they perceive to be ethical issues.

In order for a person to be autonomous it is usually considered necessary for her to be essentially self-determining, to be in control of her destiny. Autonomy is thus assumed to be desirable. Indeed it is taken to be a necessity of life by all but the most compliant people.

In most literature in medical ethics autonomy is understood primarily to involve 'personal wants' (Understanding B). On this view if a person has autonomy, and is permitted to be autonomous, then it must follow that her wishes will be respected. But this simple understanding of autonomy confuses different ideas. It is not adequate to grasp its full depth of meaning.

There are at least three different theories about the general nature of *autonomy*. It is helpful to list them.

Autonomy as a single principle
On this understanding of autonomy it is held that a basic principle exists which asserts that '*the wishes and wants of individuals ought to be respected*'. Critics of the use of this supposed principle [93] point out that 'autonomy is not the only ethical imperative'. Such critics are quite correct to say that in some circumstances other considerations take precedence over the desires of individuals (for instance, if the person has irrational desires, or if the person's desires will cause harm to other people which might have been avoided), but wrong to believe that they have therefore exposed the limitations of the usefulness of the idea of autonomy. They have not, because autonomy can be thought of in a broader way. Autonomy is such a rich notion that it cannot be said to be a simple principle without a substantial devaluation.

This mistake about autonomy is common within the pages of some medical journals, particularly in papers written on 'ethics in medicine' by doctors who have no philosophical education or experience. Philosophers reading such papers might reflect that it would perhaps have been better had the writers considered their position within the Rings of Uncertainty expressed for competence before switching on the word-processor. For example, a paper in the Journal of the Royal College of General Practitioners [94] asked doctors to report what they would do, giving their reasons, in brief vignettes concerning the *control of information* and *intervention in 'unhealthy lifestyle'*. The writers of the paper chose to differentiate 'patient welfare' and 'patient autonomy' as reasons for action. In most cases neither welfare nor autonomy were given as the most important reasons for action by the responding general practitioners (the paper's readers are left to guess what on earth the more important reasons for the interventions might be!). This paper is a perfect example of the erroneous view that autonomy is a single principle. By distinguishing between *welfare* and *autonomy* the authors assume that 'autonomy' implies 'patient control of decision-making'. For those who make this assumption the only relevant issue is, 'does the principle of autonomy apply in this case'. Almost invariably it is felt to be appropriate for doctors to decide whether or not 'the principle' should hold sway in particular cases.

Autonomy as a right
The view that autonomy is a simple principle—in the medical context, *that a patient's ability to choose should be acknowledged, and that the choice he makes ought to be respected by the doctor*—has led many writers—some of whom are philosophers—to assert that autonomy is a *right*. In other words that autonomy is something which can be claimed, and which if it is not recognised, or if it is suppressed, others have a duty to permit. To assert the right to autonomy is to assert that people ought to have self-determination and ought not to be manipulated, even if others believe that this is in their best interest.

This is a plausible view of autonomy, but again it is too simple. It regards autonomy as a single type of thing (like life or property—which you either have or have not), which everyone—apart from those people whose thought processes are severely disabled for one reason or another—can and should have. Now this makes perfect fighting sense in cases where people are repressed, where human beings are not allowed self-determination and creative self-expression, and where they might be freed. In such cases to speak of the *right to autonomy* can be a powerful and emotive weapon. In these circumstances one might scream—these people have a right to autonomy! But although this may be politically effective it is impossible to demonstrate that any moral rights exist. We have many rights in law, but laws are invented. It is simply not possible to show conclusively that the things we call 'human rights' exist in any form other than human convention. We do not have an objective right to life, we merely have life. Despite volumes of writing on the subject [95], to cast argument for change in terms of rights is ultimately philosophically unhelpful. To speak of *autonomy as a right* is to do nothing more than to assert 'I believe that the ability of human beings to choose should be acknowledged and their choices respected'. However often this is said, and by however many people this is said, autonomy does not move one jot nearer to becoming an objective right. To speak of autonomy as if it is a right is to perpetuate the myth that autonomy is a single state, something that a person either has or has not, and some *thing* that can be attained or ceded.

Note   *It is true to say that if it is argued that autonomy is a quality (as is argued below), and that this quality ought to be increased, then this belief could be translated into a principle. Equally, if a duty exists to enhance this quality in people, then it might be argued that this implies a right to have one's autonomy increased. Such interpretations are possibilities, but this book has not taken such a formal philosophical path.*

Autonomy as a quality

Against the notions of *autonomy as a principle* and *autonomy as a right* there stands a richer, far more meaningful understanding. This is that autonomy is essentially a *quality*. Autonomy is not a disembodied principle or a right somehow at least partially separate from human beings—something which can be lost forever if the right is denied. Instead autonomy is an intrinsic quality of people. At its most basic, *to be autonomous is to be able to do—to be able to do anything rather than nothing*. Autonomy, thought of in this way, is a matter of degree—the better the quality of the autonomy the more a person is able to do. A person becomes able to move more extensively in her life as her level of autonomy rises.

This view of autonomy is more complicated than the other versions, and requires more detailed explanation. The remainder of this chapter is devoted to this task. By thinking of autonomy as a quality it is possible to move forward on a number of fronts. These are the most prominent; it becomes possible to:

(1)   make a clear distinction between *creating autonomy* and *respecting autonomy*.

(2)   show conclusively that 'respecting autonomy' in the sense of 'agreeing to the wishes of others' (a derivative of Understanding B) is a very weak idea without strong and persistent reference to the creation or increase of autonomy (Understanding A). When autonomy is conceived of as a basic quality essential to the human condition, but one which can be enhanced or diminished dependent upon what happens to or is done to people, then work to increase autonomy becomes work to raise the level of human possibility. More prosaically, in a medical context it may be that a doctor considers that he is abiding by the *principle of autonomy* and respecting a person's *right to autonomy* **in full** so long as he is neutral and does not place undue pressure upon the patient. It is not uncommon to hear doctors argue for a 'laissez faire' approach as indicative of sufficient regard for autonomy—'the main thing is to let the patient make up her own mind' and 'it's not always up to me to tell the patient everything about his condition—if he wants to know then he will ask'. But without offering any additional help, then this may not be enough—the patient may not have a high enough *level of autonomy*, her autonomy may not yet be of a quality good enough to enable her to exercise a reasoned choice.

(3)   list ways of enhancing autonomy and contrast these to diminishings or constrainings. It is important to recognise that the quality of autonomy can be improved or worsened by factors that are internal to a person—factors which are at least partly within the power of the individual—and by factors external to a person.

(4)   demonstrate that in health work there can be a crucial point at which efforts to *create autonomy* (Understanding A)—efforts to improve the quality of a person's autonomy by trying to enhance what that person is able to do—become secondary

to a duty to *respect autonomy* in the sense urged by talk of principles and rights (Understanding B). It becomes possible to demonstrate that an *autonomy flip* can occur, where work to create autonomy should give way to respect for autonomy.

(5) begin to consider possible solutions to a seemingly intractable dilemma. This dilemma exists whenever it is felt that it is more important to provide for a person's *welfare* (creating autonomy in line with Understanding A) than it is to respond to a person's *expressed wants* (respecting autonomy in line with Understanding B). One trivial example of this dilemma occurs when a decision is made to deny fat children sticky buns even though the children want them. Perhaps a more serious version of this dilemma confronts doctors who work with people who experience problems with illicit drug use. Should doctors provide the drugs cheaply and safely—which is what many drug users want—or should they attempt to 'detoxify' the addicts out of concern for their welfare? Which policy has most regard for autonomy?

Autonomy as a Human Quality

It is important to review the theoretical background to the view that autonomy is a quality. It is the most comprehensive view possible to take about autonomy, but this does not mean that it has limitless meaning—far from it.

The view that autonomy is a quality stems from the theory of health as *foundations for achievement* summarised in Chapter Three. It will be remembered that according to this theory work for health is concerned essentially to remove obstacles which stand in the way of the achievement of human potential. Not all obstacles can be removed solely by cutting them away. Some obstacles can be removed only through the provision of something else. For instance, ignorance is an obstacle that can be remedied only by giving factual information. Work for health, thought of in this sense, is work to enable, work to provide a stage on which to perform. The building of this stage can be thought of both as work to remove obstacles and as work to provide additional foundations for growth. In this way the provision of the stage itself can be considered to be adding to *autonomy as quality*—adding to the extent of *movement in life* possible to a person.

Consequently, this view of health cannot accommodate a description of autonomy as a principle only, or as first and foremost as a right, but must explain it as a quality. Because health is taken to be directly related to the freedom of both body and mind, rather than directly associated with freedom from disease and illness, autonomy cannot refer only to the ability of a person to obtain her specific and intended wants. According to the theory of health as *foundations*, the idea of autonomy makes full sense only when it is thought of in terms of being *able to do* in the widest sense.

Autonomy thought of as a quality must always be conceived of in degrees rather than in absolute terms. However, it is not necessarily related to the *amount* of options available. Much depends upon context. Although a physically disabled child living in poverty as part of an uncaring family or society—a child living in conditions which disadvantage him on top of his handicap, and which no-one with power has any inclination to do anything about—will have a lower level of autonomy than a physically fit, loved, exceptionally talented Eton schoolboy; it does not always follow that wealth, age, or fitness are necessarily connected to levels of autonomy. For example, a five-year-old child will not have the same range of options as a 30-year-old middle-class insurance executive—he will not usually be able to do as much as freely—but the child will still be able to exert some control in the aspects of his life which matter most to him. For instance, he will probably be able to choose which toys he plays with, and which books he reads—within a range of options. Realistically, taking account of the different contexts of the two people, their levels of autonomy—the quality of what they might do—can be said to be roughly equivalent.

Whoever we are, whatever circumstances we live under, we are all (unless permanently comatose) able to do some things—able to move freely in some areas of life—and constrained in other aspects. These constraints can be internal to us (for example, limit of talent, limit of will-power) or external (for example, restrictions created by the desires of others, no resources to allow us to travel widely).

Thus it makes good sense to see autonomy as the ability to do things, a quality almost all of us possess to some degree, and a quality which can frequently be enhanced in a great range of ways. As such it can be seen that autonomy is far more basic to human existence than the ability to obtain what one expressly wants. This insight shows that it is possible to work to increase autonomy without having to be a docile pawn in the game of another person. It is possible to work for autonomy in this broad sense *without always having to do what another person requests*. This turns out to be a very important distinction.

Creating autonomy—enhancing the human quality of doing—is basic to health care. It is possible to represent the basic ground of work for autonomy in this way. Autonomy increases as a person moves towards the right of the spectrum (Figure 6.1).

Work to create autonomy does not necessarily imply obedience to patient choice. It is true to say that the creation of real patient choice is a primary goal, but in many cases work can be undertaken to create autonomy without direct reference to this priority. For example, it may be that a doctor believes that a person's depression might be alleviated by a change in his social life (or by drug therapy, or by ECT). To a person who is withdrawn and lethargic such a change might not seem to be desirable. It may not seem to be what she wants at all. However, if the doctor feels change in the person's social life is genuinely worth trying (and the doctor would need to be able to point to evidence to support his proposal) then, in order to create autonomy, he would be justified in a range of attempts to involve the patient in group activity. Although the doctor would not be respecting personal choice in any direct way, his intent would be to enable the patient to do more, to be freer from the grip

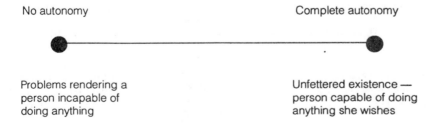

No autonomy   Complete autonomy

Problems rendering a   Unfettered existence —
person incapable of   person capable of doing
doing anything   anything she wishes

Figure 6.1

of the depression. Hand in hand with the achievement of this goal, the patient would move closer to the position where she would have a higher level of choice. This is not to say that a doctor can force a person to do something against her expressed wishes, but if there is ambivalence, then he may seek to create autonomy—but only with the specific aim of moving the person to a position on the spectrum where she is able to exercise a more fully reasoned choice (a choice free from the depression). The judgement about the point at which respecting autonomy (Understanding B) must take precedence over creating autonomy (Understanding A) is neither easy nor precisely measurable. Inevitably there will be a grey area in which there will be controversy about whether or not the *autonomy flip* (see page 126) has occurred. It is unlikely that any foolproof method exists to assist in this judgement. However, the *Autonomy Test* outlined later in this chapter can provide some practical help.

In some cases, in cases where a person is severely mentally handicapped, or where the patient is suffering from a mentally disabling illness, the notion of *respect for autonomy* may have no part to play. However, this does not mean that the issue of autonomy disappears. On the contrary, it remains as important as ever. Such a degree of handicap means that a person's life will be subject to some very severe constraints—that the person's autonomy will be of poor quality. If anything, in these cases there is all the more reason to seek avenues which enable the person, even within the severe restrictions of circumstance which surround him. When there is very little of a good thing even the smallest addition can be precious.

In very many cases, there is a clear relationship between the creation of and respect for autonomy. For instance, it is not possible for a person to express a free wish unless she knows what her situation is, unless she knows the possibilities that are open to her. So if there are three types of surgery available, and the patient thinks there is only one on offer, she may opt for it, but she will have done so with a lower level of autonomy than she might have had. She had little choice, but with the extra information she might have had, she may have made a freer choice. In this way creating autonomy (as enabling mental doing—enabling reflection in this case) can be a prerequisite for respecting autonomy (conforming with informed requests).

The fact that wishing depends upon the achievement of a certain level of being able to do—on the provision of certain conditions both for life movement and choice—is even clearer in some other cases. For example, take the case of a very frightened, anxious, nervous person entering hospital to discuss a future operation. It is possible to be in such a state of nervousness that a person is unable to think straight. The person may not even be able to comprehend properly what is being said to him,

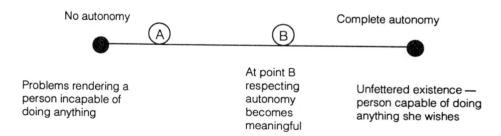

No autonomy   Complete autonomy

                    (A)   (B)

Problems rendering a   At point B
person incapable of   respecting   Unfettered existence —
doing anything   autonomy   person capable of doing
                                  becomes   anything she wishes
                                  meaningful

Figure 6.2

never mind formulate a coherent view about what to do about his circumstances and options. He may, after meeting the consultant in charge of his case, agree to a particular procedure, but since he has not been able to think at all properly it makes very little sense to say that this is what he wants. In this case, in order to have any autonomy (on Understanding B) to respect, autonomy (as being able to do—Understanding A) must be raised to a sufficient level. Looked at with reference to the continuum illustrated in Figure 6.1, the primary task of the health worker in this case is to ensure that the man moves from A to B on the spectrum (Figure 6.2).

As a general guide, the impetus of all health care interventions should be first to try to move a person as far to the right of the spectrum as possible, and secondly to move a person past point B on the spectrum at the earliest possible opportunity. Although the exact position of point B in many cases, is bound to be the subject of some controversy, and must be decided with reference to the particular facts of the case, this does not invalidate the guiding idea.

It must be said that not all doctors think of their work in this way. Those who do not cannot be said to be working for health on the terms of the theory of health as *foundations*. It is, to be sure, easier and often more efficient not to work as the first priority to move a person from A to B. For one thing the attempt to move a person is likely to be more time-consuming. But if autonomy is seriously to be asserted as an essential goal of work for health, the effort must be made.

Conditions for Autonomy

The view that autonomy is a pervasive and comprehensive stitching which holds together the best health care must be explained in as much detail as possible. Elsewhere, necessary conditions for *the creation of autonomy up to the point where it becomes a major priority to respect it*, in the absence of any overriding contraindications, have been suggested.

The conditions for autonomy

What are the basic conditions necessary for an individual to be autonomous, and how might a health service help provide these conditions?

For a person to be autonomous he or she requires three basic abilities, each of which depends upon both internal and external factors. To be autonomous it is necessary to be: (i) able to understand one's environment and circumstances; (ii) able to make (rational) choices; (iii) able to act on these choices.

All these abilities depend in part upon personal factors—for example a certain level of intelligence and perception is necessary—and in part upon factors of the wider world. For instance, a person who misperceives his personal circumstances (perhaps imagining himself to be far more—or less able—than he actually is) may be able to make choices (perhaps to pursue an unsuitable career) and may be able to act on them. But since he lacks insight and personal understanding will have a lower level of autonomy than he otherwise might. And someone serving a life sentence in prison might understand the environment, and might choose to leave it, but, as a prisoner, will not be able to act on that choice, and so will be constrained by external factors.

In order to have any of the three abilities a person must have been educated to some degree. Without education, without information, without explanations about what is happening around them no-one can begin to understand their environment. In order for people to be autonomous they must have a reasonable level of understanding of their situation, otherwise no rational choices will be possible.

There is no unanimous agreement about what rationality is but most writers in this field assent to the view that a rational choice is one in which an attainable goal is selected, and where the selection of this goal can be justified logically with reference to the prevailing external circumstances of the person. To have this ability a person needs to have adequate mental functioning, and also needs to be insulated from external pressures, such as stress, fear and depression, which might impair decision-making.

In order to be able to act on their choices, in addition to education, mental functioning, and insulation from external pressures, people also need adequate physical functioning (or assistance with physical functioning) and their personal and social circumstances need to be such that they are in a position to act on their choices. If a penniless tramp and a person earning twice the average wage for workers in a country both choose to eat three square meals a day the working person has a higher degree of autonomy because he or she is in a position to act upon that choice [96].

The basic point advanced in this quote is that certain conditions, both internal and external, must exist or be created first before a person can have enough control to be able to consider and then to say what she wants.

Anti-disease work or work for health

At this point a further insight is added to the argument that there is a persisting *category mistake* made in medicine. It is common for work against disease to disable as well as enable. Drugs have unwanted effects as well as beneficial ones. Surgery inevitably inflicts injury. Hospitalisation can be a shock, a person can feel out of control, diminished in certain ways, and she may carry this emotional trauma away with her. Indeed there are times when treating disease or perceived disease, or seeking to work against future disease through research on people, can actually move people towards the left of the spectrum rather than the right. In such cases it can be said that 'diseases' have been given too high a priority within the volatile hierarchy of human impediments. They are major problems but they are not the be all and end all of work for health, which is a broader enterprise. In such cases medicine cannot genuinely be said to be working for health unless these diminishings of autonomy cannot possibly be avoided. In health care, work to increase autonomy necessarily focuses on the individual, but not at the avoidable expense of other individuals.

Two cases

Consider the following two cases. Both involve consent, although in ways that are subtly different. *Consent* might be defined as an expressed agreement to a procedure based on a level of information which would be sufficient to satisfy the giver of that information if he were to be on the receiving end: if this is not the case then a stated decision should not be thought of as a genuine consent. Bear in mind that consent must be based ultimately in autonomy as ability to do. That is, a person must already be at a certain point on the spectrum to be able to give a consent.

CAROLE

Think about Carole, a depressed young women who is unemployed and living in an apparently close middle-class family, but one which has, below the surface, some profound tensions. Her father is terminally ill. Her behaviour consists of intermittent lethargy, drunkenness and rebellion—but overall she is dreadfully unhappy. She gets in trouble with the law. She is caught shop-lifting—a skirt from Marks and Spencer. Carole's parents decide that enough is enough, and she is persuaded to see a psychiatrist. The psychiatrist makes a diagnosis, but does not tell Carole, or her parents, his clinical conclusion. All he will say is that she has an emotional problem that she can be helped with. After a couple of weeks in hospital as a 'voluntary patient' Carole is treated as an out-patient. She is given an injection of a long lasting anti-psychotic drug (Modecate) and also another drug (Kemadrin—procyclidine) to counteract the 'parkinsonian side-effects'. She is not told what to expect by either the doctor or the nurse who administers the injection.

There are two key issues to consider in this case. *Does Carole give meaningful consent to her treatment, and in which direction is she moved along the autonomy spectrum?* These questions are crucial to the great majority of health care interventions. The answers which are given to them are of immense importance. Dependent upon what these answers are, quite different frameworks of human values can be erected. If the patient's consent is said not to matter much, if it is said that she must be cured of her supposed schizophrenia as a first priority, if her movement along the spectrum is said to be of less relevance than the need to treat, then the *category mistake* becomes pernicious.

Before considering answers to the questions in Carole's case, consider first a little more detail. The young woman is having many difficulties in her life; she is clearly at a low ebb. Carole is vulnerable. She is blamed by her family and some of her friends for causing most of her problems—'Everybody has problems, why does it always have to be you who over-reacts and makes things even worse?' For her own part she blames herself entirely for her calamity.

She desperately wants to be happier, to resolve this situation in which she feels she is drowning. She is an intelligent young woman but drifted away from school before taking her A-level exams—for which she hadn't done any work anyway. Carole has not studied or read anything other than the tabloid newspapers for the last three years: she can't be bothered to read anything else, she can't concentrate and can't see the relevance of any of it to her.

Carole becomes a 'voluntary patient' because she perceives it to be one way out. She has to do something to get out of the hole and she doesn't have many options left. In addition the pressure placed on her by her family is becoming even more unbearable. She says she agrees to the drug treatment but she has very little idea of what it will do to her, indeed whether it will benefit her in any way (although she knows that the demonstration of compliance with her family's wishes might).

The point of this example is not to criticise psychiatry (although something very close to this situation actually happened, culminating in a young person breaking out of a mental hospital through a kitchen window—to escape only to pass out and wake up after midnight covered in frost), but to show how it is possible that committing the *category mistake* can result in the diminishment of autonomy. Clearly there were many other ways in which Carole's life might have been enhanced, even if the diagnosis had been correct. When disease, or at least perceived disease, comes to be regarded as the priority, above other problems which might receive attention, then it is inevitable that other possible ways of improving a person's life are neither spotted nor pursued. Only by medicine embracing a broader theory of health will the *category mistake* be avoided more often.

EVELYN

The next example is again taken directly from life. Before it is discussed towards the end of this chapter it is presented as an exercise for self-learning or group teaching. It is important to try to recognise not only the scientific urges of research—and their dangers, but also to appreciate what it might feel like to do, and to be, a subject of research.

Exercise Seven

Research for Health?

This case is based on the experience of Evelyn Thomas and her words have been extracted from an article which appeared in The Observer. *The report of the feeling and motivation of the chief researcher are imaginary: this is deliberate, the point of these exercises is to encourage the use of the imagination—to feel as another. The justification offered by the actual researcher can be found in the* British Medical Journal [97].

This exercise describes the feelings of only two characters. The background situation is that a woman has discovered that she has been involved in clinical trials without her consent. A decision was made to have her left breast removed in order to prevent the spread of cancer. The *first trial*, which took place simultaneously in different centres around Britain, involved the testing of preventive hormonal treatment. Evelyn's treatment was compared with that of other women cancer sufferers who were receiving either no further treatment or different drugs.

The *second trial* was to test the effects of post-operative counselling. Evelyn was given no counselling whilst other patients were. Their 'psychological adjustment' was compared.

We might call the doctor Dr Alan Hughes since the position for which he argues is not unique to the actual researcher in question. The view advanced below is a paraphrased amalgam of the beliefs of several doctors. It is not intended to represent accurately the opinion of the Professor in real life.

Dr Hughes explains:

"I have been a clinical researcher and consultant surgeon for over 20 years now, and been in medicine for 10 years before that. My experience allows me to balance, in the broadest perspective, long-term human gain against possible short-term individual suffering. I would emphasise my choice of the word 'possible'. The whole

continued on next page

continued

point of research is that the answer is not known. It may turn out that the subject of a controlled trial might have benefited more from a treatment from which she was excluded, but equally she might not have done. We simply do not know for sure, which is why we need to experiment.

I know that this patient, and you could say the same of others in the past, feels hurt and perhaps abused by what I have done, but I stand by my actions and refuse to change my practice. If this patient had been informed that she was in either trial it would have rendered her inclusion scientifically invalid. We do not know the precise relationship between mental state and physical well-being, and this might have affected our results. This is particularly obvious in the case of the post-operative counselling. We were searching for very specific information, and only this information. This made it necessary for us to control as many variables as possible.

I think there are three main points to consider here: first of all each research proposal has to be passed—approved—by an ethics committee. These are committees made up of highly experienced, eminent, honourable people. Ethics committees make sure that no research proposal which is at all unethical is passed. They did not consider that I needed consent for my research because they weighed up the costs and benefits, and appreciated the considerable amount of good that potentially could be achieved by the work.

This raises the second point: if clinical research is permitted only if patients are informed, then we would not have the benefit of many scientific advances. It is vital that we advance our scientific understanding for the benefit of all future patients, and any one of us might be future patients. It must also be said that most people included in research trials do not suffer. In this case no worse treatment was given to the patient. We believed that both drug treatments were roughly equivalent.

As for the counselling trial, the patient received the highest standard of care possible from our doctors and nursing staff. It is true to say that she did not receive this particular form of specialist intervention—but at the time we had no idea whether she would benefit from it or find it to her disadvantage. In any case different people respond in different ways to all forms of medical treatment: medicine is the most uncertain of all sciences—there are always exceptions to all forms of treatment, always people who recover when they seem to have no chance of doing so.

It is also very pertinent to consider what it means to be working at this level in medicine. I cannot just sit still and rest on my laurels. I have to achieve, I have to compete. Some of my younger colleagues—men still in their forties—have published over 300 scientific papers, and I have only just over 150. I am ambitious and it is expected of me—it is an integral part of the profession that I am involved in. It is unrealistic to expect me to stop doing what so many of my peers are doing: it is part of the profession. Why should I challenge the practice, especially since I regard it to be morally quite justified."

Evelyn Thomas explains her point of view. These are her own words as reported in *The Observer* [98]:

"When I was found to have breast cancer I had high expectations of the medical profession. Like most patients I believed that doctors observed strict ethical codes. I placed absolute trust in those treating me and assumed that our relationship was based on openness and frankness. I assumed that my treatment was the only option.

continued on next page

continued

I now know that I assumed too much. Patients with breast cancer presenting themselves to my surgeon in the early 1980s had their treatment determined, without their consent, by computer randomisation. My consultant's role was to diagnose, establish eligibility for entry into clinical trials, withhold information, ensure randomisation and thereafter monitor progress. My rights to have information and to choose, and my responsibility for my own body were denied. My trust was abused. I am both deeply hurt and bitterly disappointed to have been so misused by members of the medical profession.

In retrospect, the first indication that I was in a trial came a few days after my mastectomy. The mastectomy patient in the next bed had been seen by a counsellor and given helpful information. The counsellor avoided me, and a breast prosthesis was given to me by a male fitter more used to fitting artificial limbs.

It took several years to obtain confirmation that I had been in a trial. The first trial compared post-operative counselling with no counselling: the availability of counselling was not mentioned to those randomised not to receive it.

The second trial compared three chemotherapy regimes and no treatment; the regimes were tamoxifen tablets, cyclophosphamide injections and a combination of both. Patients were again randomised—to one of the four choices—without any alternative being offered.

The administrators at the hospital have finally confirmed that I was entered into these two trials without my knowledge. Since a trial of lumpectomy versus mastectomy was also in progress at that time I suspect that I may have been in that trial since I was offered no alternative to mastectomy.

I believe that these trials were wrong for several reasons. At the very least they were unkind. It is unkind not to offer available alternatives to total breast amputation; it is unkind not to offer available counselling to all patients following breast surgery; and it is unkind not to offer to patients an alternative to cyclophosphamide with its side-effect of hair loss that is dreaded.

Withholding information about the trials may also have invalidated them. It was forgotten that patients, unlike laboratory animals, can move around and communicate with each other. Treatments are discussed and unexplained differences discovered. Inevitably these cause worry, and patients may become confused and resentful. Such feelings, and the stress produced, may be the very factors which affect health and well-being . . .

Secret trials demean patients. By depriving patients of opportunities to make informed choices, doctors appear to assume that we are unintelligent, immature and irresponsible.

Finally, I believe that such trials are unethical. I agree with the principles laid down in the Nuremburg Code for experiments on humans, which state that 'the voluntary consent of the human subject is absolutely essential' and that the person involved 'should have sufficient knowledge and comprehension of the elements of the subject matter involved as to enable him to make an understood and enlightened decision'.

Some doctors violate these ethical principles. They argue that patients cannot cope with full knowledge of their disease or uncertainties in its treatment, so that it is kinder to say nothing. Such arguments are wrong, because it is the patient or family who has to cope with an incurable and progressive disease.

continued on next page

continued

I am not arguing against scientific medical research or randomised clinical trials (RCTs). As a patient I have the most to gain from progress. As a scientist who has herself carried out physiological research on human subjects, obviously I approve of scientific methods in medicine. But RCTs must only be used with the informed consent of the participating patients. If investigators cannot convince patients that each arm of an RCT carries equal chance of risks or benefits then they must respect those patients' decisions not to participate.

My experience shows that doctors can no longer assume that secrecy in their dealings with patients can remain undetected. Yet once I did start asking questions of my consultant and hospital, the response continued to be secretive. Relevant questions about my treatment have been met with prevarication and half-truths. Approaches to various organisations such as the Community Health Council and the General Medical Council have produced little progress in getting the information, explanation and discussion that I sought. Indeed the only advice offered by the President of the GMC was that I should take legal action—a sorry reflection on the body that has a statutory duty to control the conduct of doctors.

It is good practice for such trials to be authorised before they start by the hospital's ethical committee, to see whether they are ethically acceptable. The existence of these secret trials therefore raises awkward questions about the committee's role. A letter I received last year from an administrator at the hospital said that informed consent had initially been required for the comparative trial of chemotherapy, but that after a few months the ethical committee had changed its mind. The administrator explained why:

'The reasons for this decision were that the study was being carried out on a National and European level and that other participants on the trial had not felt it appropriate to seek informed consent because of the specifically humane treatment offered in each of the arms of the study. More importantly, the experience nationally and locally was that many patients found it intensely stressful to have to face up to not only consenting to mastectomy but very shortly afterwards to have to consider the true nature of their disease and the uncertainty surrounding its management. The decision-making involved in getting informed consent was considered harmful for the welfare of some patients.'

Such reasons are not adequate to explain why the ethical committee chose to ignore the Nuremburg Code and many subsequent guidelines on the ethical conduct of research.''

Evelyn Thomas's argument was first published anonymously by the Bulletin of the Institute of Medical Ethics.

Role play/thought play

Either imagine that you are Doctor Hughes—and that you have read Evelyn's account—and a junior colleague asks you to lead a new research project which requires the diseased patients to be ignorant that they are subjects of research.

Or imagine that you are Evelyn and the information has been leaked to you by a sympathetic hospital worker that the research has been proposed, and that it has been put to Dr Hughes that he might like to become involved in it.

Where might Dr Hughes *picture* himself within the Rings?

Misunderstanding the Importance of Autonomy

The example outlined in the above exercise shows a doctor placing other values as priorities above either that of the promotion of individual autonomy or the respect for choice. There is little question that the motives of researchers in such cases are complex, and often honourable in that the work is directed towards a general increase of human welfare. But unfortunately such research is misguided because the importance of autonomy is underestimated.

In the example the researchers place the notions of not causing harm (referring to the stress that might be caused to patients by asking them if they will consent to being in a medical experiment), patient welfare (in the sense of not unnecessarily impeding the attempted clinical cure), and the well-being of future patients (who will presumably be helped by advances in the understanding of drug therapies) above that of autonomy (understood in either way). But while it is true to say that autonomy should not always be a primary drive in health care, it should not be overridden so lightly. However politically pleasing many might find the view that medicine should work essentially with communities it remains a fact that individuals suffer the disabling problems we call diseases, and that a doctor works most closely with individual patients. *The consideration of patient autonomy (in the broadest sense) must always be the starting point for a medical intervention which seeks to work for health.*

It is obvious that in the example contained in the above exercise this was not the case. Three further fundamental errors were committed by the medical professor. Briefly, the first was to think of autonomy as a single principle, the second was to commit the *category mistake* (wrongly supposing that work for health is the natural concomitant of work to counter disease), and the third was to have left Evelyn at a point unnecessarily near the left of the *autonomy spectrum* when he might—without harm to anybody else—have moved her further to the right. The professor was not working for health in this case. No genuine health work can regard people only as means, even if they are thought to be means towards greater ends.

The Autonomy Flip

Before the *Autonomy Test* is outlined both as a first step in a doctor's ethical analysis of a situation, and as a device to indicate a basic limit to medicine, it is important to consider how the different notions of create and respect autonomy might be ranked in order to guide practical interventions.

Ranking ideas within autonomy

By attempting to rank these two ideas, an apparently intractable dilemma in health care is again brought to the fore. It is this: to what extent should a person's welfare (autonomy as 'being able to do'—Understanding A) take precedence over a person's wants (autonomy as 'being able to have one's choices'—Understanding B)?

Should welfare ever take precedence over wants? All experienced health carers will be familiar with the frustration of watching a person do something to himself which the health carer thinks is foolish, or tragic, or 'bloody stupid'. Perhaps the person is eating too much or too little, smoking, drinking, engaging in unprotected sex with several partners, or injecting heroin. If the person is indulging in any of these habits, a concerned health carer might well consider that this is not good for him—that it cannot possibly be in his interest even though he thinks it is. Understandably a doctor might think that it is his task to ensure that the person changes his ways.

In such cases there can be a strong temptation for some doctors to be 'paternalistic'. In other words for doctors to give their perception of the person's welfare (often referred to as 'health') a higher priority than his choice.

Such a policy assumes this ranking of the two notions of autonomy:

FIRST: CREATE AUTONOMY

SECOND: RESPECT AUTONOMY

The expression *create autonomy* refers to basic work to enable a person (Understanding A), work to provide adequate conditions of welfare—conditions for a way of life where a person is able to realise fulfilling possibilities. For instance, educating a person about the effect of medication on her body, and ensuring that an extremely stressed person takes a rest, are both actions which would qualify as work to *create autonomy*. Work to *create autonomy* pays attention to a person's mobility in life. Work to *create autonomy* notices basic obstacles to what a person might benefit from doing, and tries to eliminate these obstacles.

Create autonomy ought to take precedence over *respect autonomy* when a person clearly faces disabling problems, and makes no objection to the doctor addressing these problems. However, at a point which varies—dependent upon circumstances and the individuals concerned—the two notions 'flip over' like this:

FIRST: RESPECT AUTONOMY

SECOND: CREATE AUTONOMY

The ultimate aim of work to *create autonomy* is to move a person to a position where she is so unfettered that she is able to exercise an informed choice about what she would like, and be able to get it. It is self evident that,

> 'Education for health is work for wholeness. It is not just to do with physical functioning, it is at least equally to do with the mental life of a person . . . work for health in its full and proper sense is work towards laying the foundations for full human flourishing.' [99]

Human beings are distinguished from most animals by our facility to think—to reflect, to introspect, to plan our actions. Not to pay particular attention to this human asset when working for health would be absurd. Choice must be a priority in health care.

The central ethical problem in health care occurs when the carer wants to carry on *creating autonomy* (as welfare), whilst the subject believes that he has reached a level of autonomy sufficient to permit a reasoned choice, and he wants his *autonomy respected*. This may mean that the subject wishes to have further autonomy created, but in a way which is unacceptable to the doctor.

Consider a case from practice. Take the example of a person who is said to be 'abusing heroin'. Whilst the notion of *create autonomy* is ranked first, the health worker can justifiably seek to push the person to the right of the spectrum. So, if the drug taker seeks help whilst intoxicated, then the health worker might offer facilities for treatment, might educate about the risks of heroin injection, might counsel, might review the person's life circumstances to see if a changed life-style might be preferable (and possible) as an alternative to heroin-taking, might show the safest ways of injecting, and might argue for whatever point of view she believes in (so long as she does not present this as the only worthwhile possibility, so long as she does not take advantage of the person's vulnerability to put forward propaganda).

However, when the *autonomy flip* can be seen to have occurred, at the point at which *respect autonomy* comes to take precedence, then *the work to create autonomy can continue but it must always be implemented so as to take the fullest possible account of the wishes of the person who is the subject of health care*. So, if the drug taker says something to this effect, 'I have listened to all you have to say, I have learnt from you, but I do not wish to stop my habit, and I do not wish you to try to make me stop anymore', and it is clear that he has the capacity to understand and has made an informed choice, then this wish must be respected.

Of course the duty to *respect autonomy* is not absolute in all cases. For instance, it is quite inappropriate if a parent insists 'I wish to continue inflicting unnecessary suffering on my children'. Autonomy ought not to be respected if the choice will deliberately harm others, and the harm is avoidable. Equally it might be the case that the doctor has to take into account wider considerations, that to *respect individual autonomy* in all cases might be to go against what might loosely be described as the 'public interest' (perhaps if the doctor were not to report a chronic epileptic patient seen driving a car).

Neither is it an implication of a commitment to *respect autonomy* that whatever a person wishes should be provided. It does not follow necessarily that because a patient wants ampules of heroin on prescription that a doctor has a duty to oblige. But what is implied is that once choice is possible, once the human faculty of reason is present, then the doctor should not positively prevent this choice unless respecting the wish would cause harm to others, or seriously undermine the subject's welfare *and the subject does not recognise this*.

It is not being claimed that even the broadest understanding of autonomy is a panacea for all moral problems. Clearly the notion of autonomy is not sufficient to cater for all situations in which it is wished to increase health, but it is an essential starting point. In some cases reflection about the importance of autonomy can be enough to indicate the merit of a policy. The use of the *autonomy spectrum* and the *autonomy flip* can be decisive, so long as the theory of health as *foundations* is accepted as the most appropriate rationale for medical work.

Dax: an illustration of the *autonomy flip*

The case of Dax is very difficult. Dax [100] was horribly burnt, left blind and without parts of his hands. Following his accident Dax wished to die, but he did not have the means to achieve his want. His doctors decided that he should live and, after long and painful treatment, Dax did live. He chose to spend his time studying and is still alive, but speaks to 'medical ethics' audiences arguing that he should have been allowed to die.

Dax's case is illustrative of the distinction between *creating and respecting autonomy*, and of the importance of appreciating how these two notions might be ranked. In one sense the doctors *created autonomy* for Dax by healing his wounds as best as they could, and enabling him to be mobile again. Yet in terms of *respect for autonomy* they seriously dwarfed him by not allowing him his chosen course (Dax was rational and not said to be mentally ill). Without an appreciation of the distinction, and without the insight offered by the *autonomy spectrum* and the *autonomy flip* there seems to be an unresolvable paradox in Dax's case. The paradox is that Dax appears to have had his autonomy both enhanced and not enhanced at the same time. Of course it is not unusual for things to happen to us which we simultaneously welcome and do not want (being forced to think more deeply is as good an example as any of this phenomenon). But if autonomy is thought of as a single principle, or as a right, then the paradox occurs.

The paradox can be solved by ranking the two notions. *Create autonomy* should be prior but only in so far as this allows doing and moves a person into a position where she can choose as freely as possible given the prevailing circumstances. But at a certain point *respect autonomy* must take over as the primary principle—suddenly the ranking flips. This is not to say that efforts to create autonomy should cease just as soon as a person is able to express a reasoned choice. On the contrary, unless a person says 'Stop!' the enabling efforts should continue if at all possible. But thought-through 'Stop!' should mean stop.

There were many future possibilities latent in the recently injured Dax, many of which were actually created, but if autonomy is to be respected in health care it was incorrect—it was an invocation of *the category mistake* in medicine—to seek to create future physical autonomy (Understanding A—being able to do) in Dax in opposition to his reasoned wish. Doctors have wishes too, but it is the patient who is treated. Ultimately the patient's wants take precedence over those of the doctor, particularly if they are negative wants—'leave me alone!'. In other words, there comes a point (which is often a clear point), where the cost—in terms of personal liberty—is so great that there is no longer any health justification for efforts to *create autonomy*.

An over-emphasis on the *creation of autonomy* as the only priority might have far-reaching social implications—beyond an obsession with health as the antithesis of morbidity into a form of authoritarianism where all risks which might produce morbidity and mortality could be outlawed.

The Autonomy Test

The Autonomy Test applies only to health care and only to individuals.

In the arena of urgent practice, images and models may seem little more than a diversion from reality. Models and decision-making tools require time to think through and to apply, and this time simply is not available to most doctors. If it is not to remain an optimistic hope that doctors might incorporate the notion of work for health into their medical practice, then something more immediately applicable is needed. On very many occasions in medical work decisions have to be made quickly, even though there are no simple rules available. What is required in these circumstances is a 'litmus test', a speedy way of obtaining a provisional indication about whether a proposed course of action ought to go ahead or not, or if it ought to be modified.

Although many decisions in medical work are made within the wide grey area where a number of reasonable possibilities can be found competing for precedence, some policies can be said to be clearly wrong. It is in its ability to help expose these cases that the *Autonomy Test* is of most value. The *Autonomy Test* adds a clear limit to the other types of limit to medical practice suggested by the description of the Rings of Uncertainty. In addition, by helping to clarify options for creative progress, by focusing on practical ways of moving a person from left to right along the *autonomy spectrum*, the *Autonomy Test* can have a role even in cases where decision-making falls within the grey area.

What is the Autonomy Test?

In one sense the *Autonomy Test* is a very basic means of checking the appropriateness of plans, and of 'brainstorming' for better possibilities for care. In another sense, although it may appear to be simple common sense, the *Autonomy Test* is one end-point of a major piece of applied philosophy. The *Autonomy Test* is one result of a distillation of a complicated, systematic account of the nature of health. As a result, to use it is to concede a great many implicit assumptions, some of which have been outlined earlier in this book and stated as the evolving conclusions (see [101], [102], [103] for the many other assumptions). Those who find the *Autonomy Test* useful should be aware of the assumptions they are borrowing. Of particular importance are the following assumptions:

(1)   Work for health is work to liberate enhancing physical and mental potential in individual human beings, so long as this causes no avoidable harm to other human beings.
(2)   That although disease can be an obstacle to the achievement of human potential, it is only one sort of obstacle in an indefinite range of possibilities, and not necessarily the most significant.
(3)   That medicine has committed a 'category mistake' by assuming that work against disease must by definition always be work for health. If the intervention does not seek to move the person to the right of the *autonomy spectrum*, or at least leave him where he is, then it is not genuine health work.
(4)   That autonomy is not essentially a single principle, or a right, but a quality which as it grows can blossom from mere unrestricted moving to a clear and decisive expression of a person's wishes.

CAVEAT EMPTOR!

The Autonomy Test—Annotated

The *Autonomy Test* consists of a number of simple questions, and requires a doctor simply to list various possibilities.

ONE

Will physical or mental autonomy not be increased when it might have been? Will it be diminished in any way?

This is a very demanding question. Only rarely in the context of medical interventions will it be possible honestly to answer NO to this question. It is very strict. The question requires that if a drug is prescribed with 'side effects' which diminish, or a person has to stay in hospital, then the response must at this stage be YES. If there is doubt about whether or not an intervention is one which acts to diminish then, if possible, seek the opinion of the subject.

If the answer is genuinely NO then go to six. If the answer is YES, or if there is any possibility that it might be YES because a factor has been overlooked, then go to TWO.

TWO

List the way(s) in which autonomy will be increased and the way(s) in which autonomy will be diminished by the proposed action:

Increases in Autonomy   Diminishings of Autonomy

Note: At this point it is inevitable that there will be disagreement about what things count as increases (enablings) and what as decreases of autonomy (diminishings). It is likely that there will be particular debate over the question of long-term and short-term autonomy. Some will take the view that although autonomy (either in the sense of being able to have wishes fulfilled, or in the sense of being able to move unfettered) is diminished in the short term, this is justified by the probable long-term increase. (This position is sometimes asserted when people are detained—in their perceived best interests—under the Mental Health Act 1983).

continued on next page

continued

THREE

Are each of these diminishings absolutely necessary?

If NO, then STOP.

Reconsider the proposed action. Consider a fresh policy.

If YES, then go to

FOUR

Will these diminishings have the effect of increasing the autonomy of the patient (according to either Understanding A or B) in the future?

If NO, then STOP. Reconsider the proposed action. Consider a policy which might work for health instead.

If YES, then go to

FIVE

Are the patient's reasoned wishes being overridden?

If NO, and the intent is to move the person to the right of the *autonomy spectrum* as soon as possible, then proceed to SIX.

If YES, then either STOP—the *category mistake* will be committed if disease is challenged at the expense of human choice—or show how this overriding of reasoned wants can be justified in another way. Possible justifications might include:

(1) The individual's wishes will harm me or others unnecessarily.
(2) The individual is reasoning erroneously—he may be thinking illogically—he may be deriving false conclusions, or he may have false beliefs (but, if so, then an attempt must be made to move him as soon as possible to the point where the *autonomy flip* can occur).

Note: *At this point in the* Autonomy Test *it is very important to bear in mind the distinction between physical autonomy—the freedom that a person has to live without physical obstruction—and mental autonomy—the freedom that a person has to make decisions and act on them. It is usual for short-term physical autonomy to be decreased in health care in order to increase long-term physical autonomy—restraining an arm in*

continued on next page

continued

a sling, or prescribing drugs which cause drowsiness in order to cure infections, or injuring a person during surgery: all these are reductions in short-term physical mobility. So long as these diminishings are not imposed against a person's wishes, they are not problematic. But here the insidiousness of the category mistake becomes truly apparent. Although it is a genuine mistake which implies no intent to harm, the mistake can be dangerous. It is one thing to stop a broken leg moving by slapping plaster of paris around it, yet quite another to prevent a person acting on her choice to drink 'too much' or to have 'too many boyfriends', by classifying her as ill and administering long-lasting tranquillisers. The reduction of mental autonomy, even in the short term with the goal of promoting long-term gain, is far harder to justify in the case of any rational person [104] (whether child or adult) who can understand the implications of what she proposes to do.

Justifications have been attempted, but they smack of the miserliness of spirit—just as a financial miser will be forever saving, waiting just a little longer until he spends. For example, it has been argued [105] that breaking a confidence (in other words not respecting a person's choice) is justified so long as this results in greater autonomy for that person in the long term. But it is hard to see the purpose of this. If the person is in a position to choose, then he should be permitted this. Otherwise, on the next occasion that the person with the power to deny choice disagrees with that choice, she will be able to justify its denial by saying that the patient is not yet autonomous enough.

What such an argument basically says is this: although you do have the capacity to choose for yourself, either you are making the wrong choice deliberately, or you cannot see that by choosing this choice you are shutting a great many doors that would otherwise be open to you. Thus, for the sake of your future capacity to choose— which should be as great as possible—I override your present capacity—and I do it for your sake.

Naturally many kind and experienced people do pursue policies such as this with those they feel could benefit from their 'hidden' support. However, it is always open to such well-meaning closet paternalists to explain in the fullest possible terms why they believe that the other person is making a mistake. There is the danger that since there is no theoretical cut-off point—no binding rule to tell the paternalist when he has gone too far, or continued for too long—that he will, using exactly the same justification time and time again, continue to override personal choice.

The Autonomy Test is clear on this. To satisfy the Autonomy Test the flip should occur just as soon as the person can weigh up the problem, review the options, and assess the implications. A free society does not wait until some ideal inspired moment—people must be free to make mistakes.

SIX

Consider the list of the ways in which autonomy might be increased (the ways in which latent enhancing human potentials might be made actual). Decide, if at all possible in partnership with the patient, the order of priority in which this list of possible potentials might be achieved.

Weigh these against any potential costs.

SEVEN

Once decided and agreed—initiate proposed action.

The Autonomy Test—Unannotated

ONE

Will physical or mental autonomy not be increased when it might have been? Will it be diminished in any way?

If the answer is genuinely NO, then go to SIX. If the answer is YES, or if there is any possibility that it might be YES because a factor has been overlooked, then go to TWO.

TWO

List the way(s) in which autonomy will be increased and the way(s) in which autonomy will be diminished by the proposed action:

Increases in Autonomy   **Diminishings of Autonomy**

THREE

Are each of these diminishings absolutely necessary?

If NO then STOP.

Reconsider the proposed action. Consider a fresh policy.

If YES, then go to

FOUR

Will these diminishings have the effect of increasing the autonomy (according to either Understanding A or B) of the patient in the future?

continued on next page

continued

If NO then STOP. Reconsider the proposed action. Consider a policy which might work for health.

If YES then go to

FIVE

Are the patient's reasoned wishes being overridden?

If NO, and the intent is to move the person to the right of the *autonomy spectrum* as soon as possible, then proceed to SIX.

If YES, then either STOP—the *category mistake* will be committed if disease is challenged at the expense of human choice—or show how this overriding of reasoned wants can be justified in another way. Go to SIX.

SIX

Consider the list of the ways in which autonomy might be increased (the ways in which latent enhancing human potentials might be made actual). Decide, if at all possible in partnership with the patient, the order of priority in which this list of possible potentials might be achieved.

Weigh these against any potential costs.

SEVEN

Once decided and agreed—initiate proposed action.

Applying the Autonomy Test

Although the *Autonomy Test* is crude and open to interpretation, it is, nevertheless, a guideline that some doctors might choose to adopt. It is enlightening to apply the test to various cases. There is no need to go into detailed ethical analysis of these cases since the *Autonomy Test* makes no claims to depth—it is a litmus test, it is a traffic light: Should I stop or should I go?

The Sidaway Case

The Sidaway Case was introduced in an earlier chapter (page 33). The dispute centred around a patient, Mrs Sidaway, who was partially paralysed as a result of an operation to relieve pain in her shoulder. She claimed that she had not been informed of the risk of damage to her spinal cord which in fact materialised, and if she had known this that she would not have consented to the operation. She sued her consultant for negligence.

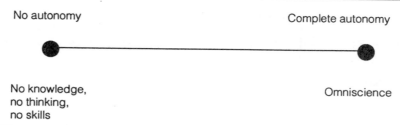

No autonomy   Complete autonomy

No knowledge,   Omniscience
no thinking,
no skills

Figure 6.3

The Sidaway Case lends itself to presentation first by means of a version of the *autonomy spectrum* (Figure 6.3).

Mrs Sidaway argued that her consent was not informed, and so not valid, since she did not know of the roughly 1% risk of damage to her spinal cord. If the bald spectrum (Figure 6.3) is taken and her position on it is considered, it might be placed somewhere towards the middle of it (Figure 6.4). It would be entirely correct to place her consultant considerably further to the right than Mrs Sidaway. The most basic question to address is this, 'Would it have been possible to create more autonomy?'. Alternatively, 'Could Mrs Sidaway have been moved further to the right of the spectrum?', or 'Could the gap between Mrs Sidaway's position and Mr Falconer's position have been narrowed?' The bald spectrum might then look something like Figure 6.4.

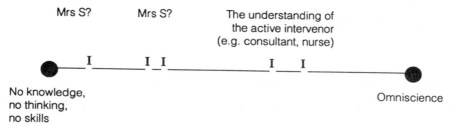

Mrs S?   Mrs S?   The understanding of
                                the active intervenor
                                (e.g. consultant, nurse)

No knowledge,   Omniscience
no thinking,
no skills

Figure 6.4

It is not possible to be precise about the positions of the various people on an ungraded scale, but what needs critical attention in the Sidaway case is the substantial gap between the level of understanding of Mrs Sidaway (who was to undergo the operation) and the level of understanding of the consultant (who was to perform it). Howard Brody, an American doctor and specialist in medical ethics, has suggested that *transparency* ought to be a guide in cases where autonomy and consent are at issue. He writes.

'The Transparency Standard

I propose the transparency standard as a means to operationalize the best features of the conversation model in medical practice. According to this standard, adequate informed consent is obtained when a reasonably informed patient is allowed to participate in the medical decision to the extent that patient wishes. In turn 'reasonably informed' consists of two features: (1) the physician discloses the basis on which the pro-posed treatment, or alternative possible treatments, have been chosen; and (2) the patient is allowed to ask questions suggested by the disclosure of the physician's reasoning and those questions are answered to the patient's satisfaction.

According to the transparency model, the key to reasonable disclosure is not adherence to existing standards of other practitioners, nor is it adherence to a list of risks that a hypothetical reasonable patient would want to know. Instead, disclosure is adequate when the physician's basic thinking has been rendered transparent to the patient. If the physician arrives at a recommended therapeutic or diagnostic intervention only after carefully examining a list of risks and benefits, then rendering the physician's thinking transparent requires that those risks and benefits be detailed for the patient. If the physician's thinking has not followed that route but has reached its conclusion by other considerations, then what needs to be disclosed to the patient is accordingly different. Essentially, the transparency standard is to engage in the typical patient-management thought process, only to do it out loud in language understandable to the patient.' [106]

Brody's request hardly seems unreasonable. All he is asking is that where there is uncertainty it should be shared absolutely between doctor and patient. If Brody's article were to be shown to a person accustomed to openness in his everyday dealings he would most likely be very surprised that Brody felt it necessary to write it. It is being suggested only that the doctor reveals his reasoning process to the person who has by far the most interest in the outcome. But this is not the climate in which medicine is generally conducted at present in either Britain or America. In Britain what counts officially as 'proper health care' is defined in law by the 'reasonable doctor'.

There is an argument that Mrs Sidaway would have been too frightened to have her operation if she had known of the 1% risk of paralysis. But this must be dismissed as an example of the *category mistake*. Given this the *Autonomy Test* is unequivocal. It shatters the Bolam Test, the test which respects only the views of 'a responsible body of medical opinion'. This test has been widely criticised, particularly by those who campaign for civil liberties and patient rights. But the law has not been changed either by the Courts or by Parliament. One reason for this might have been the absence of a workable alternative based in theory which respects the interests of both doctors and patients. This reason can no longer apply. Although the *Autonomy Test* must be interpreted, and where there is interpretation there will always be disagreement, the same can be said of any test in the uncertain world of health care. It certainly applies to the Bolam Test. However, the wording of the *Autonomy Test* is precise enough to permit clear decisions in many cases. In addition, the *Autonomy Test* rests upon a detailed body of philosophical reasoning, reasoning which is demonstrably more profound than that found in the relevant legal judgements. In order for the *Autonomy Test* to be used appropriately and honestly it must be applied according to the underpinning theory. Whenever it is not applied correctly it will be possible to show where it offends against the theory. What truly matters in health care is not what different bodies of medical opinion—and a few judges—think, but the extent to which fulfilling possibilities for living are created.

Consider how the *Autonomy Test* might have been applied to the case of Mrs Sidaway.

The Test Applied—Mrs Sidaway

ONE

Will physical or mental autonomy not be increased when it might have been? Will it be diminished in any way?

Answer Yes. Mrs Sidaway clearly might have been told more. Since the basic inspiration of health work can be shown to be the removal of obstacles to enhancing human potential, not only work against disease and illness, then it follows that health care must seek always to increase levels of autonomy (on either understanding). The speculation by a consultant that a patient might be so frightened to hear of the risk of an operation that she would not go ahead with it, and that this would be against her best interest, is fundamentally flawed. Firstly, unless the patient is given the information, there can be no convincing evidence that she will do one thing rather than another. Secondly, unless she is given the information *she will not be able to say* whether she will do one thing rather than another. Her level of autonomy will inevitably be less than it would be with the information, unless it can be proven that this information will render the person insane or irrational!

In addition, the view that fear would impede her reasoning process assumes that to be frightened is always to be irrational. This is a ludicrous assumption. When I am told that it is likely that a severe hurricane will occur over my town, and that this will bring with it a 1% risk of death or terrible injury if I do not stay in my cellar, then I will be frightened. I will also decide to stay in the cellar. However, if I discovered that 'Fat Baby' and 'Aslan' (two of my cats) were trapped outside in the storm, I might take the risk in order to rescue them. At least I would have some idea of my chances: the hurricane would be an external force acting to reduce the level of my autonomy, while my knowledge of the risk would be a force acting to raise the level.

Go to TWO

TWO

List the way(s) in which autonomy will be increased and the way(s) in which autonomy will be diminished by the proposed action.

For the purposes of the test the 'proposed action' will be taken to be 'to inform Mrs Sidaway of the general risks but not of the risk of damage to her spinal cord'.

continued on next page

continued

Increases in Autonomy
Understanding of the general
purpose of the operation

Opportunity to agree to an operation
which might create future physical
autonomy for Mrs Sidaway

Diminishing of Autonomy
Where she might have had an
understanding of the full reasoning
process of the consultant, she was
allowed only partial, and so misleading, information

THREE

Is this diminishing absolutely necessary?

Answer   NO.

So STOP. Reconsider the proposed action. Consider a fresh policy.

The *Autonomy Test* can be applied with good effect to many examples in medical work. For instance, if the example of Carole (page 121) is put to the *Autonomy Test* there is again a clear result.

The Test Applied—Carole

ONE

Will physical or mental autonomy not be increased when it might have been? Will it be diminished in any way?

Answer   Yes, unequivocally. Carole is an intelligent and able girl, yet she does not have enough information about her diagnosis and her treatment. Perhaps even more importantly no work is being done to help her *picture* what is happening to her, to help her conceive of the set of unfortunate circumstances which currently surround her—to help her map out her world. Carole desperately needs to recognise that all her problems are not her fault, that failure is just one map out of several possibilities, and that all maps have routes into each other—we can and will all fail at some things.

TWO

List the way(s) in which autonomy will be increased and the way(s) in which autonomy will be diminished by the proposed action.

In the case of Carole there have been a series of actions which have dwarfed her unnecessarily. Consider the effect of applying the *Autonomy Test* prior to drug therapy.

continued on next page

continued

Increases in Autonomy	Diminishings in Autonomy
	(Note: *not increasing autonomy where it would be possible to do so is taken to be diminishing*)
Possible alleviation of psychotic symptoms	*Things done to Carole without her understanding*
	Family not involved in any therapy
	No counselling—no picturing for Carole
	No attempt to help Carole to find a purpose in her life

THREE

Are each of these diminishings absolutely necessary?

Answer   No. Reconsider the proposed action. Consider a fresh policy.

Exercise Eight

Apply the *Autonomy Test* to the example highlighted by Evelyn Thomas, outlined on page 122. Address this proposal: it is proposed by Dr Hughes to carry out an identical research programme on human subjects. Consider your answers with reference to one of the potential subjects, Pauline Johnson.

Comment

Some doctors might find fault with these simplistic analyses. Certainly it is possible to enter into more complex moral reasoning, and to reflect on finer detail. But this is not the purpose of the *Autonomy Test*. Its purpose is twofold: to provide a *way in* for those doctors who wish to embark on deeper ethical analysis, and to illuminate clearly one limit to medical activity (demarcating legitimate medical activity is a central purpose of this book). It might be argued by those who think that each example used is clear bad practice that a test is irrelevant—that the *Autonomy Test* is hardly necessary to detect lousy medicine. But none of the examples can be said to be obviously bad practice. They did not seem to be so to the doctors and judges involved.

The Limitation of the *Autonomy Test*

It has to be acknowledged that there is much that the *Autonomy Test* cannot do. There are many cases where what counts as an increase or a decrease in autonomy is too open to interpretation for the test to be decisive. To resolve such cases, a more extensive ethical analysis is necessary, although the *Autonomy Test* will hardly ever be entirely redundant.

For instance, consider the following difficult case:

'LAW REPORT

Sterilisation of mental patient not unlawful

A sterilisation operation on a mentally disabled adult patient is not unlawful by reason only of the patient's inability to consent if it is carried out in the best interests of the patient.

The facts

F., who was born in 1953, has the verbal capacity of a two year old and the general mental capacity of a four to five year old. She has been a voluntary in-patient at a hospital since 1967, where she has formed a sexual relationship with a male mental patient. The evidence was that she had physical enjoyment from sexual intercourse with him and that she was not being sexually molested.

F. has the fertility of any other woman of her age, and her mother applied for a declaration that it would be lawful for F. to be sterilised, notwithstanding that she was incapable of consenting. Mr Justice Scott-Baker granted the declaration (Guardian Law Report December 3 1988). The Official Solicitor, who was given leave to intervene, appealed.

The decision

Lord Donaldson referred to the case of Re B[1988]AC199 in which the House of Lords held that in the case of a mentally handicapped minor the court could, acting in its wardship jurisdiction, consent to the sterilisation of the minor if it was in her best interests. This raised the stark issue of whether the law treated adults who suffered from a disability differently, and on one view less favourably, than it treated children suffering from a similar disability. In the absence of consent all, or almost all, medical and surgical treatment of an adult is unlawful, however beneficial such treatment might be.

F.'s disability was such that she would never be mentally competent to appreciate the issues involved and to consent to sterilisation or to any medical treatment. The court had no power either under the *parens patriae* jurisdiction or under any statutory jurisdiction to dispense with F.'s consent or to give consent on her behalf.

The common law right of body inviolability save with consent was subject to two exceptions: first, emergency medical treatment, and second, physical contacts which are inevitable or at least are a usual feature of everyday life, such as the jostling on public transport, or generally acceptable standards of conduct. A doctor faced with an unconscious accident patient is lawfully entitled and probably bound to carry out such treatment as is necessary to safeguard the patient's life and health, although the patient is in no position to consent.

It would therefore not be surprising if the common law rule were subject to a further qualification in relation to those who by reason of disability are unable to consent. There is a clear and logical connection between the position of an adult who through an accident is temporarily deprived of the power of consent—the emergency treatment case—and the case of an adult who through permanent disability is equally unable to consent. The difference is largely, although not entirely, one of scale.

But the law should not regard adults as permanent emergency cases. In an emergency a doctor had little time but in this case the doctor had more time, and far more was required of him.

The test which the court did, and the reasonable adult should, apply was, 'what course of action is best calculated to promote my true welfare and interests'. What constituted true welfare and interests often gave rise to very difficult questions, but that did not affect the validity of the test . . .

Lord Justice Neill said the answer lay in considering the public interest. Provided that the operation was necessary within properly defined limits and appropriate safeguards were prescribed, there was no reason in principle why a patient who could not give consent should be deprived of the right to receive the treatment required.

'Necessary' in that context meant that which a general body of medical opinion in the particular specialty would consider to be in the best interests of the patient in order to maintain his health and secure his well being. Unanimity was not required, but it should be possible to say of an operation which was necessary in the relevant sense that it would be unreasonable in the opinion of most experts in the field not to make the operation available to the patient.

Lord Justice Butler-Sloss concurred.

The appeal was dismissed, and leave was granted to appeal to the House of Lords.' [107]

The problem for the *Autonomy Test* (which is similar to, but more specific, than the 'best interest test', and does not rely solely upon the views of 'a general body of medical opinion' but on thought-through theory) is that the *autonomy flip* can never occur. F. will never be able to have a sufficient level of autonomy created for her to enable her to consider her situation, and to express a wish.

The judges decided to apply a 'best interests test', but what one person might consider to be in her 'best interests', another might not. For example, a critic of the judgement argued,

'There are a number of deeply disturbing features about this case. It is not clear that the court had the jurisdiction to make the order that it did. And it is not clear that the order made was legally correct. To equate the sterilisation operation, as the judge did, with the extraction of a tooth, the repair of a hernia or the administration of an injection, fails to recognise the enormity of the invasion and injury which the proposed sterilisation represents. It fails to distinguish between the obvious therapeutic advantages in the supposed analogies and the dubious benefits which sterilisation offers. And it fails to acknowledge that sterilisation involves major abdominal surgery requiring general anaesthesia . . .

As troubling, however are the assumptions being made about the sexuality of women with a mental handicap, the risks to which pregnancy exposes them, and the response of courts to the interests of what the judge in one place calls 'mental defectives'.' [108]

For the judges and for the author of the article the list of increases and diminishings would not be the same. A judgement has to be made about who gives the most appropriate list in terms of the creation of autonomy in F., and this is not finally empirically decidable. An analysis deeper than the *Autonomy Test* is required for this, but at least the *Autonomy Test* offers guidance in setting limits, and compels the listing of possibilities.

Clearly there is a difficulty with the ranking of *dwarfings*. Since a dwarfing must be avoided, unless to do it will prevent a worse dwarfing, it must be possible to state in general terms how one thing is worse than another. But how can subjective preferences be assessed in an objective way? Often this cannot be done—people's preferences are not the same [109]. In such cases, the only way forward is to find out, in individual context, what the person wants. This is where the *autonomy flip* is useful—and where one must respect the liberty of other people. Where the *autonomy flip* cannot occur, then great care must be taken that clearly avoidable dwarfings do not happen—and this judgement must rest on a deeper analysis and weighing of the various potential and probable harms that might come about or be avoided.

Conclusion

Clearly it would be wrong to say that in all medical interventions the total inspiration is always the creation of individual autonomy (deceit in research, unnecessary paternalism, and poor communication is presently a fact of some medical life). However, at least it can be said that avoidable dwarfings should not occur. A significant element in any true health care intervention will be to lessen impediment and to create power in the person who is being cared for. On many occasions in medical care it will be inevitable that some dwarfing—some diminishing, some limiting of what might have been—must and will be carried out. Often this dwarfing will be done in the interest of long-term good. For instance, when a person is given chemotherapy for a cancerous growth then she will feel nauseous, and may vomit repeatedly, and she will probably lose her body hair. Naturally, this increased physical distress will also be emotionally upsetting. Clearly, the person who is treated in this way will be dwarfed. She will be dwarfed physically and mentally, and she will have her short-term autonomy decreased because she will be temporarily substantially disabled by the drug therapy. The question is: How, if at all, can this dwarfing be justified in the terms of work for health as foundations?

The only justification for this sort of dwarfing is:

(1) if there is no alternative course of action (preferred by the patient) which will be less dwarfing; and
(2) if the likely consequences of the dwarfing are an increase in autonomy in the long term acceptable to the knowledgeable patient.

The key question—which this book is attempting finally to resolve—is this: Is it essentially work for health which is the inspiration of medicine, or is the goal of medicine essentially the study and cure of disease? There is a difference in these targets. The former is demonstrably more fundamental than the latter.

The difference is this: on reflection it is apparent that the study, cure and prevention of disease cannot be a basic drive because it still remains meaningful to ask—*for what reason do you study disease?* Whereas—when the question is asked without reference to the specific desires of individuals—it makes no sense at all to ask *for what reason do you attempt to make more enhancing potentials actual in human beings than there otherwise would be?*

Part III

A Framework for Growth

Chapter Seven

The Reasonable Doctor

Introduction

Medicine is a technical subject which, because it always works directly with people (rather than atoms, or bricks, or girders), inevitably has aspects which go beyond the technical. How best should I communicate this information? Should I tell this man's wife of his condition? Should I spend time with Veronica, even though it means not spending time with Jacqueline? Ought I listen to Brian, as a Samaritan would, or should I concern myself only with clinical problems? What count as clinical problems? When does undereating become a disease rather than a matter of aesthetics? When does rigorous attention to personal hygiene, or a strong sense of 'house-pride', stop being admirable and become an obsession? When does an obsession become a legitimate subject for medical intervention? When should I treat a disease with all the pharmaceutical armoury I have at my disposal, and when should I work solely to alleviate pain?

There are countless questions facing doctors which cannot be dealt with purely by science, purely by hypothesis formulation and testing, purely by the rigorous application of standard methodologies. There are countless cases in medicine where, although caring is needed, it is quite inappropriate rigorously and religiously to generate hypotheses. In such cases deeper and more extensive reasoning strategies are obviously necessary.

It is in the area of general uncertainty—uncertainty of interpretation, of self, of communication, of resources, of ethics, and of law that doctors require general problem-solving abilities. And above this doctors need the *perspective of curiosity*. The best doctors develop a constantly critical attitude, a constant questioning, in order to deal best with the broader difficulties of life which confront them.

It is not the purpose of this analysis to offer algorithms, or decision trees, or precise methodologies for dealing with these uncertainties—or to propose detailed syllabi for medical schools. There is no such thing as 'the ideal undergraduate curriculum'. To propose such a thing would not only be naive, but would be alien to the spirit of this analysis which is to give pause for thought, rather than to prescribe. However, this is not to say that any combination of subjects and any teaching method is as good as any other. On the contrary, it is possible to reach some consensus on the necessary qualities of good doctors, and this picture of the 'reasonable doctor' can help provide the pattern for an adequate programme of medical education.

The main purpose of this chapter is to consider the requirements for the 'reasonable doctor', and then to propose a basic framework within which medical students and practising doctors might best learn the skills of more than one discipline, and might best cultivate critical attitudes.

The Basic Need to Be Able to Distinguish
Types and Levels of Uncertainty

It is indisputable that medicine operates in the context of various uncertainties. Given this it is essential—a prerequisite for good practice—that students of medicine find or are shown ways of deciding, at least roughly, at which level of uncertainty they are operating, and which type of uncertainty is central to a particular case (is the uncertainty basically clinical, or legal, or ethical—or must a more complex interrelationship of uncertainties be unravelled?). Any method of medical education—and there are many—must set itself this task above all others. There is great potential danger in teaching high levels of technical competence whilst giving the impression that during every future application of these skills there will be only one kind of uncertainty to worry about, and that often the intervention will be close to certainty. The reality of intervening so intimately in other people's lives is not like this.

It is not unfair to say that present medical education does not always adopt this enlightened general perspective. A study of the syllabi of British medical schools reveals an almost unrelieved emphasis on basic science in the years prior to clinical training, and an apparently obsessive focus on the diagnosis and treatment of acute and chronic disease in hospital settings: most students find it impossible to resist the belief that the key to the best medicine is fast and accurate diagnosis, followed by the swiftest and most clinically efficient treatment. But is this all there is to medicine?

Here are two recent comments on the subject. They are by no means the last word on medical education, but they represent roughly the beliefs of many people concerned to offer useful teaching in medicine.

'In 1982 Henry Silver wrote in *JAMA* about his experiences at Denver medical school. He described seeing keen 'eager beaver' freshmen who could not wait to start on the arduous lifelong task of being a doctor and he also noted the few months it took for them to become cynical, dejected, frightened and depressed. He was a paediatrician and he thought of similar changes that he had seen in children placed in foster homes. He realised that if he had seen such changes in young children he would be concerned that something terrible had been done to them. He knew about child abuse and he wondered whether some students might be abused after entering the foster home of the medical school . . .

Unfortunately, much of our learning at medical school does not adhere to any conventional educational models. Education at its best requires active participation and questioning, with a development of the individual's potential. Goals and aims are set and the student approaches each test or exam with a positive desire to find areas of strength and weakness and to improve on deficiencies.

Not so in medicine where the instruction is didactic and uninviting of criticism. The models in current use seem to be the 'sponge', soaking up and regurgitating large volumes of information, 'the watch me', which requires a sense of mimicry, and the 'deep end' approach, which tests bravery and risk taking . . .

It is not difficult to imagine medicine as a boarding school. After a few years in the kindergarten the students proceed to the main house in the big building, working hard, fetching and carrying, doing the menial tasks as instructed by their superiors. Many are bullied by the older boys who consider these fags to be no more than servants. The house is kept in order by the consultant prefects and professorial head boys, with the school fees handled by some distant well-meaning board of governors. Survival in the boarding school depends on acceptance of the rules and a desire for a good end-of-term report or reference. Caning and fisticuffs are frowned on since the threat of a poor end-of-term report is usually sufficient motivation for most fags to comply and keep quiet.' [110]

Try as one might, by scouring the pages of *Medical Education* or *Medical Teacher* it does not seem possible to find an article which praises, argues for, or attempts to justify the perpetuation of the present system. But it persists—apparently impervious to anything other than the most minor tinkerings of reform—even in the face of vigorous pleas and campaigns for considered revision. Here, for example, is a recent declaration on the subject.

'The Edinburgh Declaration

Thousands suffer and die every day from diseases which are preventable, curable or self-inflicted and millions have no ready access to health care of any kind. Such facts have produced a mounting concern in medical education about equity in health care, the humane delivery of health services, and the cost to society.

This concern has gathered momentum from national and regional debates that have involved large numbers of individuals from many levels of medical education and health services in most countries of the world, and has been brought into sharp focus by Conference theme papers which address basic issues faced by these groups. It also reflects the convictions of a growing number of medical teachers and medical students, medical doctors and other health professionals and the general public around the globe.

The steady forward march of medicine is mainly the fruit of the research which sustains it, and a century of scientific research continues to bring rich rewards; but man needs more than science alone, and it is to meeting the needs of the human race as a whole, and of the whole person, that medical educators must now address themselves.

The aim of medical education is to produce doctors who will promote the health of all people—not merely deliver curative services to those who can afford it, or those for whom it is readily available. That aim is not being realized in many places despite the enormous progress that has been made during this century in the biomedical sciences. This problem is not new, but prior efforts to introduce greater social awareness into academic medical schools have not been notably successful.

These views indicate that many of the improvements can be achieved by actions within the medical school itself, namely to:

(1) enlarge the range of settings in which educational programmes are conducted, to include all health resources of the community, not hospitals alone.
(2) ensure continuity of learning throughout life by shifting emphasis from the didactic methods so widespread now to self-directed and independent study as well as tutorial methods.
(3) build both curriculum and examinations systems to ensure the achievement of professional competence and social values, not merely the retention and recall of information.
(4) ensure that curriculum content reflects national health priorities and the availability of affordable resources.
(5) train teachers as educators, not content experts alone, and reward excellence in this field as fully as excellence in biomedical research or clinical practice.

(6) complement instruction about the management of patients with increased emphasis about promotion of health and prevention of disease.

(7) integrate education in science and education in practice using problem-solving in clinical and community settings as a base for learning.

(8) in the selection of medical students employ methods that go beyond intellectual ability and academic achievement, to include measures of personal qualities.

Other improvements require wider involvement.

(1) Encourage and facilitate co-operation between the Ministries of Health, Ministries of Education, community health services and other relevant bodies in joint policy development, programme planning, implementation and review.

(2) Ensure admission policies that match the numbers of students trained with national needs for doctors.

(3) Increase the opportunity for joint learning, research and service with other health and health related professions.

Reform of medical education requires more than agreement; it requires a widespread commitment to action, vigorous leadership and political will. In some settings financial support will inevitably be required, but we believe that much can be achieved by a redefinition of priorities, and a reallocation of what is now available.

By this declaration we pledge ourselves and call on others to join us in a sustained and organised programme to alter the character of medical education so that it truly meets the defined needs of the society in which it is situated. We also pledge ourselves to create the organisational framework required for these solemn words to be translated into sustained and effective action. The stage is set; the time for action is upon us.'

World Conference on Medical Education of the World
Federation for Medical Education
sponsored by the
World Health Organization
United Nations Children's Fund
United Nations Development Programme
Scottish Development Agency
The City of Edinburgh
August 7–12 1988
Edinburgh

Inevitably, since it has been written by doctors who have themselves suffered at the hands of the educational system which they condemn, this declaration reveals more about the problem than it suggests practical answers. Any group of people who can write, in all seriousness, about their profession,

'. . . but man needs more than science alone, and it is to meeting the needs of the human race as a whole, and of the whole person, that medical educators must now address themselves . . .'

must be said to have a serious problem of perception. They have a quite distorted view of the power and influence of medicine: what other profession imagines it has the means, and assumes it has a right, to tackle the problems of the world?

Given such an unlimited brief, it is hardly surprising that the practical details are missing. If the medical profession is to 'meet the needs of the whole person' then it must follow that medical students must come to have a grasp of all subjects which might be useful to this end. Of course this is impossible: those who seek to change medical education must do so armed with the sense of realism which they so frequently say they value so much. The innovators must fight for reform in medical education in the clear knowledge that there are several *limits to medicine*. Only with this insight will it be possible to have a framework in which to order priorities.

Framework

There are many theories which seek to explain the continuing near inertia of British medical education. Some refer to economics (the pharmaceutical industry has a strong interest in ensuring the continuation of a system dominated by drug therapy), some to politics (it seems to be a far safer option for all political parties in Britain to express blind jingoistic faith in 'our health service' rather than wonder why it is a service possessed with the false belief that more medicine must equal more health), and some to the internal warrings of the different specialisms, each of whom are deeply dug into their respective fox-holes, and guard with rampant jealousy their allocation of teaching time.

In the face of these down-to-earth outlooks, a suggestion based in detailed philosophical thinking might seem, to some, a peculiar effort. A contribution less likely to succeed in a bid to improve medical education could hardly be imagined. However, because the theory is so well thought through, so coherent and developed—it is possible to generate workable practical proposals which can be thoroughly justified. To adopt these proposals is to carry with you the weight of philosophical analysis.

Minimum conditions for 'the reasonable doctor'

Philosophical clarification is often aimed at the discovery of *minimum necessary conditions* for the description of an event as being of a particular sort, or for the description of a particular behaviour as being legitimately of a particular kind. In this way several notable philosophers of science have attempted to distinguish between science and non-science. Just as it is not possible to distinguish absolutely between medicine and non-medicine, so the inquiry into the demarcation of science eventually exposed an area of permanent controversy [111]. However, it is possible to say that certain conditions are necessary for a practice at least to qualify as a candidate for the title 'scientific'. For instance, it can be agreed that in order for an inquiry to count as scientific it must be possible to define a problem in such a way that it is at least potentially empirically testable [112]. This condition rules out, as non-science, inquiries into the questions 'Does God exist?' or 'What is the moral status of a foetus?'

If a sensible framework to structure medical education in a coherent form is to be suggested then this, in turn, must be inspired by an understanding of the basic requirements for a person to be a doctor. Consequently, it is vital to propose a set of minimum conditions for the 'reasonable doctor'. This is not an original thought or endeavour. It will be recalled that this is what the legal system relies upon when it has to judge whether or not a doctor's performance has fallen below an acceptable standard. However, there is an importance difference. The courts rely upon a combination of legal precedent in cases relating to 'a duty of care', and medical opinion about what is reasonable. Whilst this is not necessarily an inadequate means of assessing appropriate standards in some contexts, it takes little or no account of the perceptions of 'lay-people', of the people who many doctors claim to seek to serve. Because of this oversight, it is not unreasonable to consider what set of minimum conditions might be preferred by people who are not doctors or legal judges. The set offered below have been derived from the various arguments advanced in this book. Before they are outlined it is worth addressing possible criticism.

Objection

It might be argued that it is virtually pointless for a single person to put forward conditions which he believes to be necessary for 'the reasonable doctor'. This objection has two elements.

(1)   One person can give only a highly subjective account of what *he* would like to see in his ideal doctor. Such an account might happen to concur with the views of some other people, but it is certain to be out of step with the views of most people. If minimum conditions for the reasonable doctor are to be advanced at all they should not be the result of the idiosyncratic philosophy of a single individual. They should at least emanate from either the deliberations of a multidisciplinary committee (which should include significant lay representation), or be derived from large-scale empirical research into the opinions of the general public.

(2)   According to one argument developed in this book—that it is inevitable that a plurality of models of medicine will exist—it is quite legitimate for many versions of medical activity to coexist. Since doctors' roles are many and varied, it follows that the minimum conditions necessary for a doctor to be described as a 'reasonable doctor' will vary dependent upon that doctor's special tasks.

Response to these potential objections

To take the first element: it is true to say that consensus over the minimum conditions for a reasonable doctor is unlikely. However, this truth also invalidates any other method of arriving at minimum conditions for the reasonable doctor. For instance, if the multidisciplinary committee were to reach meaningful consensus (a possibility which becomes increasingly unlikely in proportion to the number and diversity of the committee members), it is highly probable that other committees would generate different conclusions. It is equally probable that a survey of the general public would generate some patterns of preference [113, 114] but not a single coherent opinion—the public would not speak with one voice about this question.

However, the generation of some necessary conditions remains a worthwhile task. It is important that any profession—particularly a caring profession by its nature associated with vulnerable people, lays down some guidelines about how its workers should be equipped in order that people understand what to expect, and so that professionals and others can challenge these guidelines if they so wish. So long as these guidelines are open to informed criticism their source is not crucial. However, because the conditions offered in these pages have been generated out of an analysis of health and health care that has been carefully considered and scrutinised over several years, the conditions do stand a higher chance of being useful markers, and promoters of growth in medicine.

The thrust of the second element is that the range of legitimate practices in medicine is so wide that, short of such general dictums as 'the doctor must be caring and good at his professed skill', criteria for the reasonable doctor cannot be pinned down. If conditions are offered then, just like codes of professional practice, they will either be so general as to be open to various interpretations, or so specific that they will apply only to some doctors and not all of a highly heterogeneous profession.

However, there are already 'minimum conditions for a reasonable doctor' in operation, albeit often not explicitly stated. There are two obvious examples. The Bolam Test (page 32) states that a reasonable doctor will work in such a way as to meet current standards of practice. And this implies that there are minimum levels of knowledge, skill and behaviour below which a doctor must be said to be unreasonable. Secondly, medical students must pass numerous tests of competence during their training in order to ensure that they reach minimum levels of performance.

Both examples show that minimum conditions are in fact applied. Standard setting need not be hopelessly general. There are certain practices which are not acceptable, and which would fall below almost any standard. For example, it would be hard to disagree that a doctor who takes no notice of a patient's account of his symptoms, or who never respects the wishes of his patients, is not reasonable.

Suggested minimum conditions for 'the reasonable doctor'

(1) *A doctor should be technically competent to perform any clinical tasks he opts to undertake.*
(2) *A doctor should be technically competent to perform any non-clinical task he opts to undertake.*
(3) *A doctor should be able to identify the limits to his role in specific cases, and the limits to medical intervention in general.*
(4) *A doctor should be able to offer a theoretical justification for what he seeks to do. He must have a coherent rationale of care which he can explain to himself, and to those people whom he seeks to assist.*
(5) *A doctor should be able:*

- *to recognise that he is constantly operating within an arena of uncertainty;*
- *to identify which aspect(s) of uncertainty dominate in a particular intervention or proposed intervention;*
- *to appreciate roughly the degree of uncertainty which exists.*

Discussion of these conditions

It might seem that these conditions are very general. Where, for instance, are the more obvious specific practical recommendations? Where are the pleas that a doctor ought to be able both to understand his own values and to recognise that other people may have different values; that a doctor should be humble enough to respect the wishes of his patients, yet clear enough about his role to override expressed wants in order to create autonomy if this is the better option; that a doctor should be able to express his fallibility and share his uncertainties with his patients; and that a doctor ought to be adept at moral reasoning? These things are not specifically suggested since they are implicit within the broader proposals, and the present task is merely to generate a useful framework.

(1) **Clinical competence**   Medicine is a unique body of knowledge and its practitioners profess special skills and techniques. By definition it is essential that any reasonable doctor should have technical competence—but technical competence on its own is not enough.

(2) **Non-clinical competence**   Given that doctors commonly intervene in areas of people's lives which do not require specialist clinical knowledge, or technical skill, it is vital that they are competent to do so. At the very least, this requires doctors to have learnt about and have experience in a number of subjects which are not medical. At the very least, these subjects should include critical thinking, counselling, communication skills, ethics, history, law, economics, statistics, and social science.

(3) **Identification of limits**   Since a doctor must inevitably make non-clinical judgements, and intervene in the lives of others in ways which do not depend solely on clinical knowledge and technique, it is essential that he learns to know where to draw the line in his interventions. If he does not—if he regards every obstacle to human potential as his responsibility to tackle—then he will have failed as a doctor. No doctor can, or should be, clinician, marriage counsellor, business advisor, supporter and friend to every patient he meets. Equally he will need to be able to judge when to intervene beyond the clinical, when—even in uncertainty—he can be an efficient enabler.
    A doctor working with other people with different talents and backgrounds, but of equal value, must be clear that a major limit to his activity must be the patient herself. He should work to create autonomy in the areas in which he is most generally competent, and he should respect autonomy in other capable people.

(4) **Possession of a rationale of care**   In order to understand the most appropriate role for medicine as a discipline, and to detect the particular limits to his role in specific context, a doctor has to possess some underlying theoretical understanding of *what medicine is for*, some thoughtful perception of why he is doing what he is doing at all. There are many possible rationales. It is suggested that medicine thought of as work for health is the best and most flexible. It allows doctors to work creatively in both clinical and non-clinical contexts, and sets clear limits beyond which they should not seek to assist.

(5) **Recognition of uncertainty**   By understanding that medicine is saturated with uncertainty a doctor will be constantly inquisitive, critical of the information he is given, and critical of his own judgements and actions; unlikely to jump to instant conclusions; and likely to seek advice from others—from any source (whether patients, nurses, doctors, alternative healers, philosophers, economists)—as soon as he feels that he is beginning to edge more deeply into uncertainty. The doctor is far less likely to be constantly narrowly focused, constantly applying standard patterns of treatment to unique individuals in unique contexts.

How can these minimum conditions be created?

It must be stressed that these minimum conditions should not be thought to be optional, nor are some more important than others. Each is required in order for a person to be described as a 'reasonable doctor'. Technical competence is the most obvious condition, but technical competence in the absence of any one of the other conditions is not enough for balance, not sufficient for the 'reasonable doctor'. Unless it is adequate for doctors to be virtual automatons, following technical rules to the letter—never communicating with patients—then they must possess more than technical ability.

Consider a doctor who clearly is technically competent, but has no view about why this competence is worthwhile. In other words, a doctor who does not possess the other conditions. Without these, without a clear view about the rationale of his work, he will find it impossible to decide logically what to do in situations where the best form of intervention is not clear-cut. It will not be enough merely to have a sketchy view about this rationale. The doctor's theory about what medicine is for will need to be reasonably developed. For example, if the doctor's answer to the question 'What's medicine for?' is only something like 'to fight disease', then he will find himself in difficulty. If he takes this view he will be totally unequipped to deal with cases where it is unclear whether a condition is a disease or not—for instance, if he is faced with someone defined as an alcoholic. He will be unable to justify interventions in a person's life which although helpful cannot be shown to have direct pay-offs in terms of disease elimination.

Each condition is essential, but how can this set of conditions be created?

One answer: medical education structured
by the Rings of Uncertainty

Medical education tends to overemphasise the clinical aspects of care at the expense of the non-clinical. For example, in 1989 undergraduates at Liverpool University received only 10 hours basic tuition in ethics in 5 years, which is 10 hours more than the students received prior to 1989. In addition to this marked imbalance, medical education is notorious for its lack of integration. The various disciplines tend to consider themselves to be quasi-autonomous mini-kingdoms with some laws of their own. To have the various teachers working *within* each Department understand what their specialist colleagues are doing—to know the content of each other's lectures—is rare. To have all the various specialisms communicate—so as not to repeat material, and so as to develop some continuing educational threads is virtually unheard of.

The Rings of Uncertainty might be used to change this situation. Although medical teachers would need compulsory in-service training to be able to use them, even if only in a minor way, *this would be the only immediate change necessary*. The basic content of the existing syllabus, and the teaching time allocated, could—at least for the time being—remain exactly as it is. Any threat to the status and credibility of the different disciplines and their advocates would be minimal.

How would this reform work?

Recall the Rings set in rigid form, with equidistance between the segments (Figure 7.1).

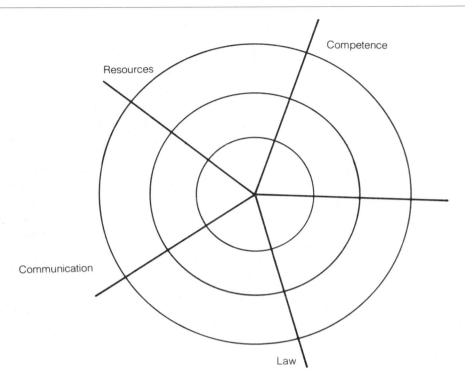

Figure 7.1

It would be possible to add other segments to this basic model. For example, cost-effectiveness or risk might be useful inclusions. Equally, it could be argued that less segments might be used. For instance, law might be subsumed under ethics, or communication might be omitted, its meaning covered by the competence segment. However, while the choice of segment rests in personal judgement, the five categories in Figure 7.1 are recommended as the most effective way to promote constructive reflection about a doctor's role.

A Basic Programme

The reform to medical education would make use of the rings in the following way:

As medical students enter medical school they would immediately be introduced to the Rings of Uncertainty. They would be told that the challenge of medicine is to deal with uncertainty as effectively as possible, and that to do this much knowledge and skill is required—both of medical science and of other disciplines which study human behaviour and thinking. Each segment of the Rings would be discussed, and its relevance demonstrated by the use of appropriate clinical examples. The teachers leading the introductory sessions would, by discussing cases from their own experience, show how a doctor could think of himself as standing within different levels for each segment.

Each student would receive a carefully written introductory booklet which would explain much academic information which students might find useful throughout their period at university. The students would be advised to keep their booklets safe since they might wish to refer to them at any point during their student days. Their attention would be drawn to the opening section covering the Rings where they would be explained carefully, and where further illustrative examples from medical practice would be given.

If all the teaching staff of a medical school could be convinced of the value of taking the Rings seriously as an educational device, and would be prepared to reinforce the booklet material, then—far from seeming cranky or perverse—the Rings would have real credibility. Students would become used to them, and expect to meet them from time to time during their education. At a stroke, this would be a dramatic unifying force, pulling together seemingly disparate subjects within a strong common framework. Preclinical teaching should also attempt to make use of these Rings. If the basic science subjects cannot find a way to use the Rings creatively then this should not necessarily be thought to be an unfavourable reflection on the Rings. On the contrary, questions might be raised about the value of spending so much time teaching pure material to people who are destined to practise medicine in uncertainty.

The Rings used by each training block

Each teaching department should prepare its course material with reference to the model of the Rings of Uncertainty. The medical educators should start with a picture of the Rings with the hands set at neutral—just as the students encountered them in the introductory lectures. The medical teachers might then do two things with the Rings.

Firstly, in the introductory lecture to the teaching of their specialism they should prepare slides to show how the dividing lines might be moved—both apart and together—dependent upon the importance of any particular segment. Naturally different proportions will be chosen by the different specialisms: for example, the 'surgical firm' might have up to 85% of the Rings devoted to technical competence, although with significant proportions devoted to the other four segments—perhaps as in Figure 7.2 (which does not accurately reflect this percentage).

Obstetrics and gynaecology might have an even larger portion devoted to law and ethics, while general practice might have a more proportional balance of all segments, perhaps with particular emphasis on communication. It should be crystal clear by this stage of the book that it will be a very limited, unimaginative and *unrealistic* programme of teaching which claims to operate within only one segment.

Secondly, thoughtful medical teachers might be able to use the Rings creatively within their specialist teaching programme, although some might be content to use them only to help structure a strong educational programme. For example, since the Rings can be graded as they move out from near certainty towards greater and greater uncertainty it is possible to discuss current issues, developments and controversies within any specialism using the Rings as a specific educational tool. Thus, a good teacher of transplant surgery might, for instance, lead a discussion session on organ transplantation in the context of scarce resources, making full use of the Rings. The teacher might suggest a number of scenarios, and use a number of positions within

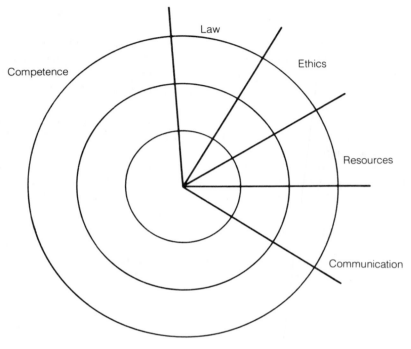

Figure 7.2

the Rings, in order to encourage students to generate a range of suggestions as to how to deal with the various uncertainties. A good teacher of general practice might ask students to imagine how they would deal with a patient's case (where the problem is revealed step by step and the student asked to comment at each stage—rather as a problem would appear in real-life), not only with reference to the practical management and the important non-clinical features, but also by raising and pressing the issue of positioning within the Rings. The students might be asked to use their imaginations to consider where they would see themselves standing within the Rings. The inevitable disagreements which would emerge about individual placings would provide invaluable discussion material.

Over all specialisms a far broader range of questions, questions not normally felt to be part of mainstream medical practice might make much more sense, and be easier to ask with the help of the Rings. The type of questions which form the backbone of this book might become commonplace. For example, '*What is the goal of your medical work in this case*' '*What is your proper role here?*' '*At what point must you call a halt to your endeavours?*' '*In what areas are you best able to help?*' '*In what proportion should you provide help in the various areas in which you are competent?*'

Benefits

There are a number of immediate benefits which might be enjoyed as a result of the application of the model of the Rings. These are:

(1) It will be essential to provide in-service education for medical teachers who will not have experienced this form of critical thinking. Naturally there will be some resistance, but it is to be expected that many teachers will welcome the opportunity to explore new methods, and perhaps to consider other models of education for the first time.

(2) The model will provide a constant theme to guide medical students throughout their education.

(3) The permanent reference to levels of uncertainty and ways of dealing with them will allow students to appreciate the reality of medical practice during their training, rather than be exposed to the misleading focus of precise hospital work.

(4) The use of the model will be a significant factor in the validation and spread of 'non-clinical' subjects such as ethics and communication.

(5) The presence of the Rings will make it far more likely that non-clinical teachers will be accepted by both medical teachers and medical students.

(6) The use of the model will allow experimentation with different educational methods by clinical teachers.

(7) Students will feel more confident that their education has been structured with a view to continuity and integration.

(8) Whilst students will be taught much accurate medical information, material which perhaps comes close to the truth, they will not believe this information to be absolutely true. They will appreciate that the history of medicine shows that 'knowledge' is constantly refuted or revised as situations change. Information will not be thought of in terms of blacks and whites, but in terms of degrees of uncertainty. With this new emphasis students will inevitably be less inclined to be passive receptors and acceptors. Since they will not believe that they are learning 'the gospel truth' they will feel far more free to be critical.

(9) If medical students are critical of nothing else, as they gain experience they will at least learn to be critical of the space devoted to particular segments over others. It is to be expected that observant students will soon appreciate how open to interpretation the Rings are, not least because they will see how different teachers and specialisms use them. This, more than anything else, will reveal the extent of uncertainty in medicine.

The curriculum

What might the medical curriculum look like? Although it would not be impossible to come up with a proposal for an 'ideal undergraduate syllabus' this would not be a productive exercise. It would serve only to create dispute—about hours, about organisation, about neglected subjects—which would detract from the main message of this book for medical education. This is that change must come from medicine itself—through the negotiated efforts of medical teachers and students, rather than be imposed externally.

Numerous innovations and experiments in medical education have been designed and suggested. These include courses in the behavioural sciences and humanities, increased exposure to out-patient medical care, Faculty development, alterations in grading systems designed to reduce competition, the restructuring and reordering of curricula to integrate the basic sciences with patient care, and (in America) some limited effort to combine training of medical and nursing students [115].

All these changes might well be candidates for a reformed programme of medical school teaching. In addition, a brave medical school might experiment with teaching students in community settings, introducing students to patients from the first day of their education, confining students to hospital beds and wheelchairs for short spells (not as punishment, but as an aid to their imagination), and teaching medical students alongside students of other Faculties.

Conclusion

A simple model for change in medical education has been offered. It is based upon an analysis of medicine as work for health which has generated a set of minimum conditions for the 'reasonable doctor'. If these conditions are indeed accepted as being reasonable expectations then serious thought must be given to their creation. The most direct method must be to develop medical education. The Rings of Uncertainty might be adapted to make this possible. If this is done it will not be necessary to overthrow existing practices and replace them with radical new programmes. On the contrary, the beauty of the Rings is that they can enhance medical education without major surgery.

The use of the Rings of Uncertainty does not have implications only for medical education. They might offer significant help with communication between the various health care professions, and between these professions and the subjects of care. This application of the model is discussed in the next chapter.

Chapter Eight

Implications for other Health Workers

There are many implications of the thesis advanced in this book. Some are practical, and some are theoretical in so far as they affect the ways in which health workers are able to think about, and justify, what they do. Several of these implications have been discussed in the preceding pages. In addition it is important to explain how the Rings of Uncertainty might be used to enhance understanding and communication between the various professions whose task it is to provide health care. In a book which is more concerned to raise awareness of new possibilities than to describe detailed policy it is not appropriate to draw out detailed Rings of Uncertainty for all health workers. Members of the various professions might well prefer to experiment for themselves. However, there is advantage in demonstrating how the Rings of Uncertainty for two other types of health-care professional—nurses and health educators—might be used in constructive conversation with doctors about roles and limits.

In order for any conversation to take place those who are to speak must share the same framework of meaning. Consequently, in the ensuing analysis it is assumed that all those who might participate in discussion take the same general view of health (a narrow one in this case). It is also assumed, for the sake of convenience, that the doctors, nurses and health educators involved adopt the same wording for the Rings. This may not be the case in reality, but there is no reason in principle why the wording of the Rings, fully expressed, should not be interpreted to suit the particular purposes of each profession, or of individual patients.

Recall the image of the Rings of Uncertainty fully expressed (Figure 8.1).

What might this image mean for a nurse? Just as the image of the Rings of Uncertainty might spark off a wide variety of pictures and ideas in the minds of doctors, so it might inspire a wealth of intellectual conceiving in the nurse. For instance, for her, the *resources* segment might not relate primarily to hospital budgets, but to staff levels and the availability of materials on her ward which might be used to ensure reasonable standards of hygiene and dignity. She might regard the *communication* segment to be a particularly valued specialism—something which she believes some doctors wrongly disparage. And she might well feel that there is an element of competition between nurses and doctors over the *technical competence* segment—recalling more than one occasion where, tactfully, she had to suggest an appropriate dosage of a drug to a junior doctor.

The Rings of Uncertainty must have meaning added to them by the people who wish to use them. They exist to be interpreted. Although such freedom may not appeal

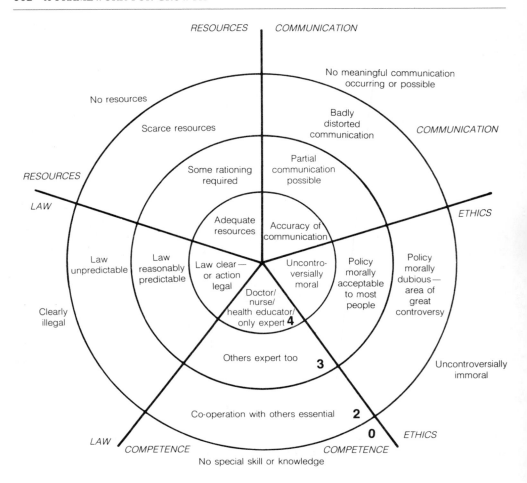

Figure 8.1

to those who feel most at home with the quantifiable aspects of life, the Rings do provide an excellent framework for communication since they set some clear limits (words cannot mean anything one wants them to mean) but at the same time permit negotiation.

They might be used creatively either in a teaching session involving a mixed group of health-care professionals (unfortunately all too rare an educational experience in the territorial world of professional health care), or in a situation in life where negotiation is to take place. Consider this latter case. Here it may be necessary to suspend belief about the balance of power held by the various negotiators—assume that the doctors, nurses and health educators are to conduct the conversation as equals!

Reflect on the following situation. Representatives of doctors, nurses and health educators are meeting to discuss the provision of health care in a new Health Centre which is to be designed from scratch in an inner city area. A philosopher had also been included on the working group but could not accept that the design of the Health Centre had to begin from a base seated in medicine and the provision of services directly set against disease. Despite several attempts to convince the planning team that there is no necessary relationship between disease and health, and despite the team's almost continuous assertions of agreement with this position, the philosopher saw no practical evidence of enlightened thinking—only of limited ideology. Consequently the philosopher resigned, explaining that he had done so because of the sad lack of realism displayed by the committee. He went off to build bridges elsewhere.

The remaining members of the planning team decide that the most fruitful way to design the new centre is not to start with a discussion of the question, 'What services ought there to be?' but with debate about the *extent of the professional roles of the staff of the centre.* They decide to make use of the Rings of Uncertainty (which are only as good as the imagination of those who use them!). The planning team decide that each of the three professions should, for a range of categories—including treatment, prevention, education, and screening—place markers within the Rings of Uncertainty (drawn on transparent acetates) according to their perceived positions—according to their perceived competencies and circumstances.

KEY

O = Nurse's *picturing*
X = Doctor's *picturing*
Z = Health Educator's *picturing*

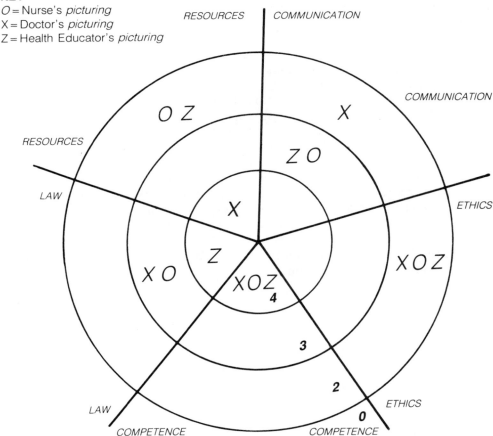

Figure 8.2

Figure 8.2 shows the pattern that emerged for the category of *prevention*.

Despite the fact that the blueprint for a Health Centre which might eventually be produced at the end of the negotiation process will not be as imaginative or comprehensive as the philosopher would have liked (for instance, it will not include an adult-education centre, an advice bureau staffed by lawyers and welfare workers, nor will it include a public bar), the use of the Rings in this way can be a stimulating device for open, honest discussion about the provision of caring services. A number of events will occur.

(1)   The acetates completed by each specialism will be arranged together, so that they superimpose.
(2)   There will be a period of surprise during which each of the groups will think about the placings of the others, and about what this means about their perceptions of their roles.
(3)   After this initial period of adjustment there must be lengthy clarification—using specific practical examples of cases which might well be encountered—of what each group understands by the wording of the segments.
(4)   Following this it will be necessary for each group, having arrived at a consensus— or something closer to it than before—to review their original placings, and draw up fresh charts.
(5)   At this point the heavy negotiation can begin in earnest. If, for instance, each of the groups considers that it sits in exactly the same place in terms of technical competence for *preventive activity* (albeit over a different span of activities), then it becomes both possible and desirable to reassess the allocation of roles. Tradition may be shown not to be the best model for innovation. It may turn out that the health educators, most of whom will have been trained in teaching and communication methods, will have the most time left in the developing scheme of things—and so be best placed in terms of *resources* to take over the previously accepted role of doctors and nurses in this area. It may then fall to this group to take charge of the design of the entire prevention programme for the Centre.
(6)   The process of negotiation might then move to other areas, the outcome of which might eventually feedback to affect the area of prevention.

The process would be enormously complex, but undertaken in this way might generate some refreshing solutions and vital insights.

Chapter Nine

Conclusion

General Liberation

The intention of this book has been to offer general ideas to assist practical progress in medicine. The various insights and models which have been put forward have implications for all health workers, not only doctors of medicine. However, the primary aim has been to generate frameworks to enable clinicians to practice with a clearer appreciation of the extent of and limits to their roles.

The most obvious place to launch the suggested changes of structure is within medical education. If students of medicine can be helped to appreciate the presence of uncertainty in medicine at the earliest possible stage, then they will be better equipped both to have a realistic view of their own learning process, and to offer a good standard of care throughout their careers. Through changes in medical education students will come to recognise the need for a broader set of knowledge and skills than that created by more traditional teaching.

More is implied by the argument of this book than change only to educational theory and practice. Other practical effects are inevitable and must be recognised in tandem with the benefits of the implementation of the ideas outlined in this book. Although the *Rings of Uncertainty* and the *Autonomy Test* might be brought into mainstream medical education without wholesale alteration to the content of teaching as it is now, nevertheless their introduction would bring with it a change of spirit.

Slowly medicine would come to be thought of in a different light. If doctors are to take on the task of liberating themselves by acknowledging the need to explore fresh attitudes and approaches to their subject, then they become vulnerable. In effect, by confessing that medicine should seek conceptual innovation clinicians relinquish some of the power associated with an image of a science aiming for certainty. Doctors will find it necessary to admit that they need the assistance of several non-clinical disciplines in order to grow as a profession which can work for health rather than solely against disease. Such an admission is hardly shameful, but will require brave and confident innovators.

In a culture where all professions have become intensely specialised, work for health in a broad sense is possible only through collaboration. At the very least the permanent presence is required in medical schools of experts in philosophy, history, law, education, communication, economics, social science, statistics, and demography—as equals in every sense with clinicians. Through this recruitment of new talent medicine will reap a reward in increase of knowledge, skill and insight—at the cost of the loss of a veneer of certainty.

Currently, at least in the academic world, it seems that the various disciplines—including those listed above—exist in their own particular rarefied atmospheres.

Each academic specialism not only has its own theoretical terrain to defend, but has a unique culture such that there can be only limited understanding and sharing between disciplines. What this means in practice is that the various academic professions often consider issues from their own special perspective without necessarily ever taking account of the views of the other professions. Interdisciplinary meetings to discuss issues of mutual interest are the exception rather than the rule. As a result of this reluctance—and inability—to share it is not uncommon for entirely irrelevant academic work to be produced.

By involving many professions in the endeavour to transmit a broad practical theory of work for health, it becomes more likely that useful academic research will take place. So-called applied philosophy, or applied economics, or applied social science, might become truly applied given the benefit of a proper appreciation of the reality of the circumstances of medicine. For example, over the past few years, a sizeable body of literature has emerged about 'health-measurement' [115]. Academics from several disciplines have added their thoughts to the debate, but with little appreciation of the perspectives of their colleagues from other subjects, or—apart from the medics—of the reality of practice. The Quality Adjusted Life Year (QALY) [116] has been suggested as a workable tool for assessing whether a person ought to receive a treatment or not. Or if the treatment is a scarce resource, whether patient A or patient B should receive it. Philosophers and economists have argued at length about the morality of the QALY, but they have mostly done so from a hypothetical perspective, often mistaking their distorted image of medical reality for the real thing. Perhaps in an ideal world when a kidney becomes available from a cadaver it would be possible to reflect carefully—using sophisticated measuring devices if necessary—about which of all the possible recipients might gain the most benefit from it. But, like it or not, the real world is not like this. What actually happens when kidneys become available from a cadaver is that one is offered to the United Kingdom Transplant Service (UKTS) for computerised matching to the ideal recipient, while the other is retained by the hospital in possession of the body in order that the local transplant unit might make use of it, almost certainly by offering it to a less well-matched person. This reality seriously undermines a great many of the theoretical debates about health measurement [117]. It is not that the debates themselves are uninteresting, but that they could be far better applied with knowledge of the reality of the situation.

By learning about the reality of medical practice non-clinicians can gain stimulus and inspiration in their work—experience gained from another area of life can feed into their own form of inquiry. This experience can have several benefits. It can offer a challenge to mistaken or unjustified assumptions about practice; in conversations with doctors non-clinicians sometimes have to explain the value of their work (and vice versa)—a process which can, at times, be both salutary and enlightening; theories encountered in a medical environment can strike chords and spark off unexpected chains of thought; and overall there can be an appreciation of why doctors do what they do—rather than puzzlement about *how anyone might possibly be able to do that* (for instance, lack of comprehension about how a psychiatrist could detain a schizophrenic patient in hospital against his will, or how a doctor could ever justify a policy of keeping information from a patient).

This book has argued that the best medicine stems from a realistic appreciation of the reality of working to remove obstacles to people's mental and physical potentials in an environment which is steeped with a variety of uncertainties. It has explained that disease, although an important topic which in order to be properly understood requires intensive training over several years, is not an *exceptional* human problem. Disease is one of a range of states which may or may not be perceived to be a problem by human beings. There is no natural order where disease is ranked always as a more serious problem than other problems of life. As a result of this insight it becomes essential that doctors develop a view of their work which allows them to delineate their roles more precisely. This can be done by thinking of medicine as work for health, and by noting the limits on medical practice which can be derived logically from this outlook. At least some of these limits have been encapsulated by the *Rings of Uncertainty* and the *Autonomy Test*.

In a sense the theory presented in this book is quite obvious. It has a feel of being intuitively correct. It seems to be an articulation of a great many strands of opinion both within and outside medicine. When these elements are viewed separately, considered on their own, each seems almost to go without saying. But taken together they are far more powerful. If these embryonic ideas gain credence in medical circles then a crucial step towards the liberation of medicine will have been taken.

References

1. Illich, I. *Limits to Medicine*. Penguin, 1975.
2. Kennedy, I. *The Unmasking of Medicine*. Penguin, 1981.
3. Bursztajn H., Feinbloom, R., Hamm, R., Brodsky, A., *Medical Choices, Medical Chances. How Patients, Families and Physicians Can Cope With Uncertainty*. New York: Delacorte Press/Seymour Lawrence, 1981.
4. Sidaway v Board of Governors of the Bethlem Royal Hospital [1985] AC 871, [1985] 1 All ER 643.
5. Butler, N. Anorexia Nervosa: an overview. In Scott, D. (ed) *Anorexia and Bulimia Nervosa: Practical Approaches*. London: Croom Helm, 1988;3-23.
6. Palmer, R.L. *Anorexia Nervosa: A Guide for Sufferers and their Families*. Penguin, 1988.
7. Stanley, I.M. Meshtel *Trainee* 1983 (December).
8. Stanley, I.M., Heywood, P.L. Data Linked Groups: A Method for Continuing Professional Education. *Medical Education* 1983;**17**:390-394.
9. *Mental Health Act (1983)*. London: HMSO; 1983.
10. Brazier, M. *Medicine, Patients and the Law*. Penguin, 1987.
11. *Ibid.*
12. Foucault, M. *Madness and Civilisation: A History of Insanity in the Age of Reason*. London: Tavistock, 1967.
13. Rockstein, M., Sussman, M.L. *Nutrition, Longevity and Ageing*. New York: Academic Press, 1976.
14. 'Phyllis is risen'. *Guardian* 1988: August 6th.
15. Makin, P.J., Rout, U., Cooper, C.L. Job Satisfaction and Occupational Stress Among General Practitioners—a Pilot. *Journal of the Royal College of General Practitioners* 1988;**38**:303-308.
16. Hodkin, K. *Towards Earlier Diagnosis*. 5th ed. Edinburgh: Churchill Livingstone, 1985 p. 273.
17. *Ibid*, p. 344.
18. Breckenridge, A., Dollery, C.T., Parry, E.H.O. Prognosis of Treated Hypertension. Changes in Life Expectancy and Causes of Death Between 1952-1967. *Quarterly Journal of Medicine* NS 1970;**39**:411.
19. Stamler, J., Stamler, R. Intervention for the Prevention and Control of Hypertension and Atherosclerotic Diseases: United States and International Experience. *Am J Med* 1984;**76**:13-36.
20. Australian National Blood Pressure Study Management Committee. The Australian Therapeutic Trial in Mild Hypertension. *Lancet* 1980;**i**:1261-1267.
21. Multiple Risk Factor Intervention Trial: Risk Factor Changes and Mortality Results. *JAMA* 1982;**248**:1465-1476.
22. Medical Research Council Working Party. MRC Trial of Treatment of Mild Hypertension: Principal Results. *British Medical Journal* 1985;**291**:97-104.

23. Ayman, D., Goldshire, A.D. Blood Pressure Determinations by Patients with Essential Hypertension. The Differences between Clinic and Home Readings Before Treatment. *Am J Med Sci* 1940;**200**:465–474.
24. Floras, J.S., Hasson, M.O., Sever, P.S., Sleight, P. Cuff and Ambulatory Blood Pressure in Subjects with Essential Hypertension. *Lancet* 1981;**ii**:107–109.
25. Mancia, G. Methods for Assessing Blood Pressure Rates in Humans. *Hypertension* 1983; 5 suppl.**111**:5–13.
26. Pickering, T.G., Devereux, R.B. Ambulatory Monitoring of Blood Pressure as a Predictor of Cardiovascular Risk. *Am Heart J* 1987;**114**:925–928.
27. Pickering, T.G., James, G.D., Boddie, C., *et al.* How Common is White Coat Hypertension? *JAMA* 1988;**259**:225–228.
28. 1988 Hypertension Annual. London: Gower, 1988.
29. British Medical Association, *ABC of Hypertension*, BMA, London, 1981.
30. Drug and Therapeutics Bulletin. Consumers Association, October 1989.
31. Tudor-Hart. *Hypertension*. Edinburgh: Churchill Livingstone, 1980.
32. *Blacks Medical Dictionary*. 30th ed. Adam and Charles Black, London, 1974.
33. Wright, H.J., Macadom, D.B. *Clinical Thinking and Practice*. Edinburgh: Churchill Livingstone, 1979.
34. Elvebeck, L.R., Guillier, M.A., Keating, Jr., F.R. Health, Normality, and the Ghost of Gauss. *Journal of the American Medical Association* 1970;**211**:69–75.
35. Brazier, M. *Medicine, Patients and the Law*. Penguin, 1987.
36. Mason, J.K., McCall Smith, R.A. *Law and Medical Ethics*. 2nd ed. London: Butterworths, 1987.
37. Kennedy, I., Grubb, A. *Medical Law: Text and Materials*. London: Butterworths, 1989.
38. *Ibid*, pp. 376–377.
39. Brazier M. *Medicine, Patients and the Law*. Penguin, 1987;53–54.
40. Kennedy, I., Grubb, A. *Medical Law: Text and Materials*. London: Butterworths, 1989;395–396.
41. *Ibid*.
42. *Ibid*, pp. 248–249.
43. Unnamed in Caplan, A.L., Englehardt, H.T. Jr., McCartney, J.J. (eds). Concepts of Health and Disease: Interdisciplinary Perspectives. Reading, MA: Addison-Wesley Publishing Company, 1981;109/107.
44. Sedgewick in *Ibid*, pp. 120–121.
45. *Op cit*.
46. Hoffman-Axthelm, W. *History of Dentistry*. Chicago: Quintessence, 1981.
47. Engelhardt, H.T. Jr. In: Complan, A.L., Engelhardt, H.T. Jr., McCartney, J.J. (eds). Concepts of Health and Disease: Interdisciplinary Perspectives. Reading, MA: Addison-Wesley Publishing Company, 1981;266.
48. Ryle, G. *The Concept of Mind*. Penguin, 1963.
49. World Health Organisation. Constitution. Geneva: World Health Organisation, 1946.
50. Seedhouse, D.F. *Health: The Foundations for Achievement*. Chichester: John Wiley, 1986; 74–75.
51. Seedhouse, D.F. *Ethics: The Heart of Health Care*. Chichester: John Wiley, 1988;80.
52. Seedhouse, D.F. *Health: The Foundations for Achievement*. Chichester: John Wiley, 1986.
53. *Ibid*, pp. 61–62.
54. *ibid*, p. 61.
55. Teeling Smith, G. (ed). *Measuring Health: A Practical Approach*. Chichester: John Wiley, 1988.
56. Seedhouse, D.F. *Health: The Foundations for Achievement*. Chichester: John Wiley, 1986.
57. Seedhouse, D.F. *Ethics: The Heart of Health Care*. Chichester: John Wiley, 1988.
58. Turner, B.S. *Medical Power and Social Knowledge*. London: Sage Publications, 1987.

59. Childress, J. F. *Who Should Decide?: Paternalism in Health Care*. OUP, New York, 1982.
60. Freidson, E. *Profession of Medicine*. New York: Dodd, Mead and Company, 1975.
61. Illich, I. *Limits to Medicine*. Penguin, 1975.
62. Jarman, B. (ed) *Primary Care*. Oxford: Heinemann, 1988.
63. Goodman and Gillman. *Pharmacological Basis of Therapeutics*, 3rd edition, Macmillan, 1967.
64. Folb, P.I. *The Thalidomide Disaster and its Impact on Modern Medicine*. University of Cape Town, 1977.
65. Godlovitch, S., Godlovitch, R. (eds) *Animals, Men and Morals: An Enquiry into the Maltreatment of Non-humans*, London: Gollancz, 1971.
66. Goodman and Gillman. *Pharmacological Basis of Therapeutics*, 3rd edition, Macmillan, 1967.
67. Carnworth, T., Johnson, D. Psychiatric morbidity amongst spouses of patients with stroke. *Br. Med. J.*, 1987;294.
68. Pharoah, P.O.D., Harnabrook, R.W. Endemic Cretinism of Recent Onset in New Guinea. *Lancet* 1974;**ii**:1038.
69. Bailey and Loves. *Short Text Book of Surgery*.
70. Feyerabend, P. *Science in a Free Society*. London: NLB, 1978.
71. Seedhouse, D.F. *Ethics: The Heart of Health Care*. Chichester: John Wiley, 1988.
72. *Health Matters*. London: Health Matters Publications.
73. Robinson, M.B. Patient Advocacy and the Nurse: Is there a Conflict of Interest. *Nursing Forum* XXII No. 2, pp. 58–63.
74. Black, D., Townsend, P., Davidson, N. *Inequalities in Health: The Black Report*. Penguin, 1982.
75. Whitehead, M. *The Health Divide: Inequalities in Health in the 1980s*. HEC, Wembley, 1987.
76. Wilson v. Pringle [1987] QB 237, [1986] 2 All ER 440, CA.
77. Koestler, A. *Janus: A Summing Up*. London: Hutchinson, 1978.
78. *Hansard*. House of Lords 10 November 1987, cols 1350–51.
79. Bolam v Friern Hospital Management Committee [1957] 2 All ER 118 [1957] 1 WLR 582.
80. Harrison, B. *An Introduction to the Philosophy of Language*. London: Macmillan, 1979.
81. World Health Organization. *Mental Disorders: Glossary and Guide to their Classification in Accordance with the Ninth Revision of the International Classification of Diseases*. Geneva: WHO, 1980.
82. Koestler, A., Smythies, J.R. *Beyond Reductionism, New Perspectives in the Life Sciences*. Hutchinson, 1972.
83. *Gillick v West Norfolk and Wisbeck Area Health Authority* [1984] 1 All ER 365 per Woolf J; revsd [1985] 1 All ER 533, CA; revsd [1985] 3 All ER 402, HL.
84. DHSS Guidelines (H C (86) 1).
85. Brazier, M. *Medicine, Patients and the Law*. Penguin, 1987.
86. *R v. Arthur* (1981).
87. *Re B (a minor)* [1981] 1 WLR 1421.
88. Gillon, R. *Philosophical Medical Ethics*. Chichester: John Wiley, 1985.
89. HMSO (January 1989) *Working for Patients*.
90. Seedhouse, D.F. *Ethics: The Heart of Health Care*. Chichester: John Wiley, 1988.
91. Gillon, R. *Philosophical Medical Ethics*. Chichester: John Wiley, 1985.
92. Seedhouse, D.F., Cribb, A. *Changing Ideas in Health Care*. Chichester: John Wiley, 1989.
93. Baum, M., Zilkha, K., Houghton, J. *Ethics of Clinical Research: Lessons for the Future*. *BMJ* 1989;**299**:251–3.
94. Christie, R., Freer, C., Hoffmaster, C.B., Stewart, M.A. Ethical Decision Making by British General Practitioners. *Journal of the Royal College of General Practitioners* 1989;**39**:448–451.

 95. Waldron, J. (ed) *Theories of Rights*. Oxford: Oxford University Press, 1984.
 96. Seedhouse, D.F., Cribb, A. *Changing Ideas in Health Care*. Chichester: John Wiley, 1989.
 97. Baum, M., Zilkha, K., Houghton, J. *Ethics of Clinical Research: Lessons for the Future*. *BMJ* 1989;**299**:251-3. (See also: Baum, M. I didn't abuse my patients. *Observer* 1988; October 16:8.)
 98. Thomas, E. *Observer* 1988; October. (See also: Thomas, E. Informed Consent. *Lancet* 1986;**ii**:1280.)
 99. Seedhouse, D.F. *Health: The Foundations for Achievement*. Chichester: John Wiley, 1986.
100. Dax's Case. In: Kliever, L.D. (ed). *Essays in Medical Ethics and Human Meaning*. Dallas: Southern Methodist University Press, 1989.
101. Seedhouse, D.F. *Health: The Foundations for Achievement*. Chichester: John Wiley, 1986.
102. Seedhouse, D.F. *Ethics: The Heart of Health Care*. Chichester: John Wiley, 1988.
103. Seedhouse, D.F., Cribb, A. *Changing Ideas in Health Care*. Chichester: John Wiley, 1989.
104. Seedhouse, D.F. *Rationality*. (PhD thesis) Manchester: Manchester University, 1984.
105. Komrad, M.S. A Defence of Medical Paternalism. *Journal of Medical Ethics* 1983;**9**:38-44.
106. Brody, Howard. *Hastings Centre Report* September/October 1989;7-8.
107. *Guardian*, 1988: December 4th.
108. *Guardian*, 1988: December 9th.
109. Rosser, R.M., Kind, P. A Scale of Valuation of States of Illness: is there a Social Consensus? *International Journal of Epidemiology* 1978;**7**:347-357.
110. Collier, J. Medical Education as Abuse. *BMJ* 1989;**299**:1408.
111. Brown, Harold, I. *Perception, Theory and Commitment*. Chicago: University of Chicago Press, 1977.
112. Popper, K.R. *Objective Knowledge*. Oxford: Oxford University Press, 1979.
113. You and Your GP. *Which*, 1989.
114. Al-Bashir, M. *A Preliminary Study of Factors Affecting Patients Preferences for Some Aspects of General Practice*. Unpublished Thesis. Department of General Practice, Liverpool University.
115. President's Commission for the Study of Ethical Problems in Medicine and Biomedical and Behavioural Research (1982), *Making Health Care Decisions*. Vol. 1: Report.
116. Rosser, R.M., Kind, P. A scale of valuation of states of illness: is there a social consensus? *International Journal of Epidemiology* 1978; **7**:347-357.
117. Harris, J. Qualifying the value of life. *Journal of Medical Ethics* 1987;**13**:117-123.

Index